KEY TOPICS IN
RENAL MEDICINE

The KEY TOPICS Series

Advisors:

T.M. Craft *Department of Anaesthesia and Intensive Care, Royal United Hospital, Bath, UK*
C.S. Garrard *Intensive Therapy Unit, John Radcliffe Hospital, Oxford, UK*
P.M. Upton *Department of Anaesthetics, Treliske Hospital, Truro, UK*

Anaesthesia, Second Edition

Obstetrics and Gynaecology

Accident and Emergency Medicine

Paediatrics

Orthopaedic Surgery

Otolaryngology and Head and Neck Surgery

Ophthalmology

Psychiatry

General Surgery

Renal Medicine

Forthcoming titles include:

Oncology

Oral Surgery

KEY TOPICS IN
RENAL MEDICINE

C.R.V. TOMSON
MA, BM, BCh, FRCP, DM (Oxon)
Southmead Hospital, Westbury-on-Trym, Bristol, UK

W.D. PLANT
BSc, MB, MRCPI
Royal Infirmary of Edinburgh, Edinburgh, UK

βIOS
SCIENTIFIC
PUBLISHERS

© BIOS Scientific Publishers Limited, 1997

First published 1997

A CIP catalogue record for this book is available from the British Library.

ISBN 1 85996 170 3

BIOS Scientific Publishers Ltd
9 Newtec Place, Magdalen Road, Oxford OX4 1RE, UK
Tel. +44 (0)1865 726286. Fax. +44 (0)1865 246823
World Wide Web home page: http://www.Bookshop.co.uk/BIOS/

DISTRIBUTORS

Australia and New Zealand
 DA Information Services
 648 Whitehorse Road, Mitcham
 Victoria 3132

India
 Viva Books Private Limited
 4325/3 Ansari Road, Daryaganj
 New Delhi 110002

Singapore and South East Asia
 Toppan Company (S) PTE Ltd
 38 Liu Fang Road, Jurong
 Singapore 2262

USA and Canada
 BIOS Scientific Publishers
 PO Box 605, Herndon
 VA 20172-0605

Important Note from the Publisher
The information contained within this book was obtained by BIOS Scientific Publishers Ltd from sources believed by us to be reliable. However, while every effort has been made to ensure its accuracy, no responsibility for loss or injury whatsoever occasioned to any person acting or refraining from action as a result of information contained herein can be accepted by the authors or publishers.

The reader should remember that medicine is a constantly evolving science and while the authors and publishers have ensured that all dosages, applications and practices are based on current indications, there may be specific practices which differ between communities. You should always follow the guidelines laid down by the manufacturers of specific products and the relevant authorities in the country in which you are practising.

Typeset by Chandos Electronic Publishing, Stanton Harcourt, UK.
Printed by Redwood Books, Trowbridge, UK.

CONTENTS

ABBREVIATIONS

ACE	angiotensin-converting enzyme
ACEIs	angiotensin-converting enzyme inhibitors
ADH	antidiuretic hormone
ADPKD	autosomal dominant polycystic kidney disease
AIDS	acquired immunodeficiency syndrome
AIN	allergic interstitial nephritis
ANA	antinuclear antibodies
ANCA	antineutrophil cytoplasmic antibodies
ANF	antinuclear factor
APD	automated peritoneal dialysis
APTT	activated partial thromboplastin time
ARF	acute renal failure
ATN	acute tubular necrosis
BCG	Bacille Calmette-Guérin
BP	blood pressure
CAPD	continuous ambulatory peritoneal dialysis
CAVH	continuous arteriovenous haemofiltration
CAVHD	continuous arteriovenous haemodiafiltration
CBF	cerebral blood flow
CCD	cortical collecting duct
CIN	chronic interstitial nephritis
CLED	cystine lactose-deficient
CMV	cytomegalovirus
CNS	central nervous system
CPAN	classical polyarteritis nodosa
CRF	chronic renal failure
CRP	C-reactive protein
CT	computed tomography
CVVH	continuous veno-venous haemofiltration
CXR	chest X-ray
DAA	dialysis–associated amyloidosis
DI	diabetes insipidus
DIC	disseminated intravascular coagulation
DKA	diabetic ketoacidosis
DMSA	dimercaptosuccinic acid
DNA	deoxyribonucleic acid
dsDNA	double-stranded DNA
DTPA	diethylene triamine pentaacetic acid
DVT	deep-vein thrombosis
ECF	extracellular fluid

ECG	electrocardiography
EDTA	ethylenediamine tetraacetic acid
EGF	epidermal growth factor
ELISA	enzyme-linked immunosorbent assay
EM	electron microscopy
ENA	extractable nuclear antigen
ENT	ear, nose and throat
ESI	exit-site infections
ESR	erythrocyte sedimentation rate
ESRF	endstage renal failure
ESWL	extra-corporeal shock wave lithotripsy
FACS	fluorescent-activated cell sorter
FBC	full blood count
FDP	fibrin degradation products
FSGS	focal segmental glomerulosclerosis
GB3	globotriasoyl ceramide 3
GBM	glomerular basement membrane
GFR	glomerular filtration rate
GI	gastrointestinal
GN	glomerulonephritis
HBV	hepatitis B virus
HCV	hepatitis C virus
HD	haemodialysis
HDL	high-density lipoprotein
HELLP	haemolysis, elevated liver enzymes, low platelets
HFRS	haemorrhagic fever with renal syndrome
HIV	human immunodeficiency virus
HIVAN	HIV-associated nephropathy
HLA	human leucocyte antigen
HMG CoA	3-hydroxyl-3-methyl glutaryl-coenzyme A
HRS	hepato-renal syndrome
HUS	haemolytic uraemic syndrome
IDDM	insulin-dependent diabetes mellitus
IgA	immunoglobulin A
IgM	immunoglobulin M
IIF	indirect immunofluorescence
ITU	intensive therapy unit
i.v.	intravenous
IVU	intravenous urography
KHF	Korean haemorrhagic fever
KUB	Kidneys, ureter and bladder X-ray
LDH	lactate dehydrogenase
LDL	low-density lipoprotein

LVH	left ventricular hypertrophy
MAG3	mercaptoacetyl triglycine
MCD	medullary cystic disease
MCGN	mesangiocapillary glomerulonephritis
MHC	major histocompatibility complex
MPA	microscopic polyangiitis
MR	mannose resistant
MRFIT	multiple risk factor intervention trial
MRI	magnetic resonance imaging
MS	mannose sensitive
MTALH	medullary thick ascending limb of the loop of Henle
NAE	net acid excretion
NE	nephropathica endemica
NIDDM	non-insulin-dependent diabetes mellitus
NSAIDs	non-steroidal anti-inflammatory drugs
$1,25\text{-}(OH)_2D_3$	$1,25$-dihydroxy-vitamin D_3 (activated vitamin D_3)
OTC	over-the-counter
PD	peritoneal dialysis
PET	peritoneal equilibration test
PKD	polycystic kidney disease
pmp	per million population
PTH	parathyroid hormone
PTHrP	parathyroid-related peptide
PUJ	pelvi-ureteric junction
RA	rheumatoid arthritis
RAA	renin–angiotensin–aldosterone
RBC	red blood cell
rHu-EPO	recombinant human erythropoietin
RIA	radio-immune assay
ROD	renal osteodystrophy
RPF	retroperitoneal fibrosis
RPGN	rapidly progressive glomerulonephritis
RRT	renal replacement therapy
RTA	renal tubular acidosis
SAA	serum amyloid A
SAH	subarachnoid haemorrhage
SAP	serum amyloid P
SBE	subacute bacterial endocarditis
SIADH	syndrome of inappropriate ADH secretion
SIRS	systemic inflammatory response syndrome
SLE	systemic lupus erythematosus
TAE	total acid excretion

TALH	thick ascending limb of the loop of Henle
TGF	T-cell growth factor
TGF-β	transforming growth factor-β
TPN	total parenteral nutrition
TTP	thrombotic thrombocytopenic purpura
USS	ultrasound scan
UTI	urinary tract infection
VDRL	Venereal Disease Research Laboratory
VTs	verocytotoxins
VUR	vesico-ureteric reflux
vWF	von Willebrand factor
WG	Wegener's granulomatosis

PREFACE

There seems to be a widespread belief that renal disease is especially complex and conceptually difficult. Many students and non-specialist doctors view it as an intimidating topic. We believe that this is not true, and present this text as an aid to making renal medicine comprehensible, accessible and interesting. Our approach is based on experience gained from teaching this subject to a wide range of medical and paramedical staff.

We have addressed 50 topics in renal medicine. We hope that in each section the subject is presented concisely but comprehensively, combining aspects of epidemiology, pathophysiology, clinical presentation, diagnosis and management. To our knowledge, the facts presented are the most up to date available from the literature at the time of publication.

This text should provide the reader with a significant core of knowledge of the subject presented. Guidance for further reading in more extensive textbooks or reviews is provided at the end of each topic.

This book should be of particular value to those studying for postgraduate examinations, especially in medicine. It may serve as a useful, brief textbook for those working in disciplines in which renal disease is often encountered (such as urology, surgery, medicine, and anaesthesiology). We would also recommend it to general practitioners, nurses and medical students who have an interest in learning more about renal medicine.

We would like to thank our publisher, BIOS Scientific Publishers for their assistance and patience during the preparation of this text.

C.R.V. Tomson
W.D. Plant

ACID–BASE DISORDERS: GENERAL APPROACH

Acid–base disturbances occur when disease processes cause disruption of normal homeostatic mechanisms or when the acid or (more rarely) alkali burden presented exceeds the adaptive capacity of these mechanisms. Significant renal impairment is always associated with acid–base disturbance.

Normal H$^+$ homeostasis

- Normal arterial pH ranges from 7.36 to 7.42. Intracellular pH ranges from 6.40 to 7.35. pH is maintained by intracellular and extracellular buffers, and by renal and respiratory regulatory mechanisms.
- pH is $-\log_{10}$ [H$^+$]. This relationship is almost linear over the range of plasma values commonly encountered in clinical medicine. For each change of 0.1 pH unit, [H$^+$] changes by about 10 nmol/l. pH of 7.4 represents [H$^+$] of about 40 nmol/l. pH rising to 7.5 represents a drop in [H$^+$] to about 30 nmol/l. pH of 7.0 is equal to [H$^+$] of 100 nmol/l.
- Resting production of H$^+$ ions ranges from 15 000 to 25 000 mmol/day. Of this, up to 20 000 mmol/day are produced by tissue respiration and excreted as CO_2 by the lungs.
- Organic acid production accounts for 2500 mmol/day (lactic acid, hydroxybutyric acid, acetoacetic acid and free fatty acids produced by liver, muscle and adipose tissue). These organic acids are metabolized, rather than excreted, by the liver, kidneys and heart. Having a low renal threshold, ketone bodies may also be excreted by the kidney. Lactate, with a threshold of 5–10 mmol/l, exhibits little renal excretion.
- Smaller quantities of non-volatile 'fixed' acids (sulphuric and phosphoric acids) are produced from the metabolism of sulphur-containing amino acids and organic phosphates. These can only be excreted by the kidneys.
- Buffers such as haemoglobin, proteins, bi-carbonate and phosphate play a transient role in

counteracting pH changes. Ultimately all generated H^+ ions need to be excreted. The time to critical acidaemia depends upon the nature of the upset, the excretory system most impaired and the class of acid generated.

Renal control of acid excretion

- H^+ secreted into the proximal tubule binds with filtered HCO_3^-. The resultant carbonic acid is dehydrated by carbonic anhydrase to H_2O and CO_2. H_2O is excreted and CO_2 diffuses back into the blood, to be excreted by the lungs. This sequence, which is intimately associated with proximal tubule sodium reabsorption, prevents bicarbonate loss but causes no net acid excretion.
- H^+ secreted into the tubular lumen also binds with non-bicarbonate buffers such as urate, creatinine and, most importantly, phosphate. The increased production of NaH_2PO_4 contributes to net urinary acid excretion and is quantified as the 'titratable acidity'.
- Ammonia is produced in the tubular cells and diffuses into the lumen. Secreted H^+ binds with ammonia to form the ammonium ion (NH_4^+). Ammonium ions are trapped within the lumen and excreted.
- Total acid excretion (TAE) by the kidney is the sum of titratable acidity and urinary ammonium excretion. Net acid excretion (NAE) is the sum of these minus any excreted bicarbonate. NAE approximates to 1 mmol/kg/day.
- NAE is influenced by the pH, pCO_2 and potassium concentration of body fluids, by the effective circulating volume, by the action of mineralocorticoids and by the level of renal function.

Classification systems

- When NAE is less than net acid generation plus net acid ingestion then acidaemia will occur unless compensatory mechanisms exist. Acidosis is defined as a pathophysiological state wherein acidaemia will occur if left unopposed. As compensatory mechanisms usually exist, patients may be acidotic with a relatively normal plasma pH. The converse applies for alkalosis and alkalaemia.

- Acidosis due to a primary reduction in plasma bicarbonate is termed a metabolic acidosis. If due to a primary retention of carbon dioxide it is termed a respiratory acidosis. Similar definitions are used for alkaloses. Compensatory mechanisms involve the development of an opposing acid–base disturbance. For example, with metabolic acidosis partial compensation will be achieved by the development of a respiratory alkalosis.
- Metabolic acidoses are further classified by the anion gap. This is an estimate of 'unmeasured anions'. The anion gap is calculated as plasma $[Na^+] - ([Cl^-]+[HCO_3^-])$. The usual value is 12 ± 4 mmol/l.
- Metabolic alkaloses may be further classified as chloride-responsive or chloride-resistant.

Metabolic acidosis with increased anion gap

- Uraemic acidosis occurs with advanced CRF, usually when the GFR is less than 25 ml/min. There is decreased capacity to excrete the non-volatile 'fixed acids'. Although renal ammoniagenesis is increased in surviving nephrons, total excretory capacity is decreased by the absolute reduction in total functioning nephrons.
- Diabetic ketoacidosis occurs in states of relative insulin deficiency. There is increased lipolysis and release of free fatty acids by adipocytes. With an associated glucagon excess there is stimulation of the hepatic metabolism of fatty acids to ketoacids. Adrenaline, growth hormone and cortisol also promote ketogenesis.
- In starvation and chronic alcohol abuse there is accentuated hepatic ketone production and reduced plasma insulin concentration, which can also lead to ketoacidosis.
- Type A lactic acidosis occurs with tissue hypo-perfusion and hypoxia, as occurs in cardiogenic shock, sepsis, cardiorespiratory arrest, carbon monoxide poisoning and severe hypotension.

Type B lactic acidosis occurs in a heterogeneous group of conditions, including treatment/poisoning (with biguanides, ethanol, methanol, cocaine, cyanide and salicylates), thiamine deficiency, malignancy, sepsis and phaeochromocytoma. D-lactic acidosis may occur with bacterial overgrowth of the gastrointestinal tract and may not be detected by laboratory tests for the more usual L-lactic acid.

- Salicylate poisoning results in an increased anion gap due to a combination of salicylate, lactic acid and ketones. Methanol poisoning generates formic acid, formaldehyde and lactic acid.

Metabolic acidosis with normal anion gap

- Typically there has been a loss of body bicarbonate, with plasma chloride rising to compensate and maintain a normal anion gap.
- Gastrointestinal fluid losses occur in diarrhoea, through biliary and pancreatic fistulae, and when urinary diversions to the gut have been created. Bicarbonate-rich fluid, secreted into the upper GI tract by the pancreas and hepatobiliary system, is not reabsorbed lower down the GI tract.
- Urinary diversions to the sigmoid colon commonly cause metabolic acidosis. This is less common with diversions to ileal loops, unless these are obstructed.
- Renal tubular acidoses.
- Infusion of the cationic amino acids arginine and lysine.

Chloride-responsive metabolic alkalosis

- Vomiting, nasogastric suction and use of diuretics with potent chloruretic actions (loop diuretics and, to a lesser extent, thiazides) lead to loss of hydrochloric acid or chloride-rich fluid from the GI tract or kidney. This is associated with signs of ECF volume depletion. Urinary chloride concentration is low (<10 mmol/l) and potassium deficiency may coexist.
- Administration of sodium chloride solutions corrects this problem. Volume expansion is not necessary (although possibly desirable for other reasons). With resolution there is increased

bicarbonate secretion in the cortical collecting duct (CCD). This apical chloride–bicarbonate exchange requires the presence of luminal chloride in the CCD, which in turn requires an adequate GFR and adequate chloride administration.

Chloride-resistant metabolic alkalosis

- Primary retention of sodium bicarbonate by the kidney occurs in states of mineralocorticoid excess. Urinary chloride concentration is greater than 20 mmol/l. There are usually signs of ECF volume excess and hypertension. Severe potassium depletion causes a similar problem.
- Bartter's syndrome presents with a hypokalaemic, chloride-resistant metabolic alkalosis. There is frequently magnesium and sodium wasting with associated symptoms. This condition may be difficult to distinguish from surreptitious diuretic or laxative abuse – conditions more likely to cause a chloride-responsive alkalosis.

CNS control of ventilation

- Several distinct areas in the pons and medulla control involuntary respiration. The medullary chemoreceptor responds to changes in pCO_2. Peripheral receptors in the carotid bodies respond to changes in pCO_2.
- Respiratory alkalosis increases CNS lactic acid production and decreases cerebral blood flow (CBF). Respiratory acidosis slightly increases CBF. Changes in cerebrospinal fluid pH are less marked with metabolic disturbances. Metabolic alkalosis increases CBF. Metabolic acidosis decreases CBF. Acute metabolic acidosis causes a marked drop in pCO_2. This is less marked with chronic metabolic acidosis. Acute metabolic alkalosis increases pCO_2.

Respiratory acidosis

- This occurs in conditions with a primary increase in pCO_2.
- Primary failure in the CNS drive to ventilation occurs with anaesthesia, overdose, cerebral trauma and central sleep apnoea.

- Primary failure in transport of CO_2 from alveoli to atmosphere occurs with airways obstruction, restrictive disorders such as flail chest and severe pneumonitis, and neuromuscular diseases such as Guillain–Barré syndrome and myasthenic crisis.
- Primary failure of transport of CO_2 from tissues to alveoli occurs in shock and pulmonary oedema.

Respiratory alkalosis

- This occurs in conditions with a primary decrease in pCO_2.
- Increased stimulation to respiration may be central in origin due to anxiety, hyperventilation, pregnancy and neurological disease.
- Increased stimulation to respiration may be driven by tissue hypoxia with chronic high-altitude exposure, severe anaemia, pulmonary embolism and cyanotic heart disease.

Further reading

Garella S. Clinical acid/base disorders. In: Cameron JS, Davison AM, Grünfeld J-P, Kerr D, Ritz E (eds) *Oxford Textbook of Clinical Nephrology*. Oxford: Oxford University Press, 1992; 917–65.

Nairns RG, Jones ER, Townsend R, Goodkin DA, Shay RJ. Metabolic acid-base disorders: pathophysiology, classification and treatment. In: Arieff AI and DeFronzo RA (eds) *Fluid, Electrolyte and Acid-Base Disorders*. New York: Churchill Livingstone, 1985; 269–384.

Related topics of interest

Acute renal failure: general approach (p. 11)
Chronic renal failure (p. 31)
Disorders of extracellular volume (p. 54)
Drug-induced renal disease (p. 57)
Dyskalaemias (p. 63)

ACUTE RENAL FAILURE: ACUTE TUBULAR NECROSIS AND SELECTED SYNDROMES

Acute tubular necrosis (ATN) is the most common pathophysiological entity found in established acute renal failure (ARF). It usually occurs as the result of a number of nephrotoxic insults occurring simultaneously or in succession. It has an excellent prognosis for recovery if the patient survives the associated underlying medical or surgical problem.

Causes

- ATN usually results from an ischaemic renal insult, in situations such as trauma, surgery, haemorrhage, sepsis, post-partum haemorrhage and pancreatitis. Pre-existing risk factors are often found.
- Extracellular fluid (ECF) volume depletion alone tends not to cause ATN unless it is severe, protracted and occurring with other insults.
- Nephrotoxic agents such as drugs, radio-contrast agents or ethylene glycol may cause a toxic ATN, as may pigments such as myoglobin.

Pathophysiology

- Widespread necrosis of tubular cells is relatively uncommon. More usually there is loss or internalization of apical microvilli, flattening of epithelial cells and necrosis of scattered tubular cells. Cellular dysfunction rather than disintegration is more evident.
- Renal vasoconstriction is an early and central pathogenic event. Ischaemia leads to sloughing of the brush-border microvilli. Tubular swelling may interfere with tubular and vessel patency. Cellular debris from the proximal tubule may form casts in association with Tamm–Horsfall protein. These casts may obstruct the tubular lumen.
- Sublethal ischaemic injury to proximal tubular cells leads to a change in polarity, with Na^+/K^+-ATPase appearing at the apical rather than the basolateral aspect of cells. This may disrupt normal mechanisms and direction of sodium reabsorption, with reduced sodium reabsorption being a pattern frequently observed. This defect

is corrected by re-oxygenation with subsequent cellular remodelling.

- Although the kidney as a whole extracts less than 10% of the oxygen carried through it, there is an area where the balance of oxygen delivery and oxygen consumption is precarious even in normal circumstances. The thick ascending limb of the loop of Henle in the outer medulla (MTALH) is metabolically active but has a relatively low oxygen delivery. Up to 80% of delivered oxygen is extracted here. When ischaemia occurs, this area may be the first part of the kidney to suffer necrosis. Haemoconcentration can lead to erythrocyte trapping in the outer medulla, a feature not usually seen in the cortex.

- Much experimental work supports the thesis that many events may be modulated by local concentrations of calcium ions and free radicals of oxygen. This may be especially so in reperfusion injury, as may occur in renal transplantation.

Recovery from ATN

- Classically, the kidney recovers from ATN by passing through a diuretic phase, with polyuria and impairment of tubular function. Replacement of crystalloid and important ions such as K^+, Mg^{2+}, Ca^{2+} and PO_4^{2-} may be necessary to avoid fresh lesions of ATN.

- Repair involves the synthesis of many mediators, such as epidermal growth factor (EGF) and transforming growth factor-β (TGF-β). Provision of adequate nutrients and calories is important to this process.

Myoglobinuric ARF

- Muscle damage with release of myoglobin into the circulation may cause ARF with proximal ATN and pigmented casts in the distal nephron. Dipstick-positive haematuria with no red blood cells on urine microscopy is a characteristic finding, as is an elevated creatinine phosphokinase level. The urinary sodium concentration is often low.

- Causes include traumatic crush injuries and protracted coma with pressure necrosis which may follow self-poisoning. Compounds directly toxic to muscles, such as alcohol and cocaine, may be implicated. In up to 40% of cases no unequivocal cause can be identified–viral myositis, especially if due to coxsackievirus, may be important. Patients with intrinsic muscle disease are more vulnerable to rhabdomyolysis. Lipid-lowering drugs can cause this syndrome, especially in patients with CRF.
- Tubular obstruction occurs due to precipitation of myoglobin in the increasingly acidic sections of the nephron. ECF volume depletion often coexists, facilitating precipitation further.
- Early treatment of crush injury victims with a sodium bicarbonate and mannitol diuresis maintains urine flow and prevents development of ARF. The consensus is that the urine flow rate is the more important feature, with urinary alkalinization and free radical scavenging being less important.

Acute urate nephropathy

- Occurs in haematological malignancy, especially Burkitt's lymphoma, and after chemotherapy or radiotherapy when turnover of cells increases with increased nucleoprotein degradation.
- ARF can be due to obstruction of the distal tubule and collecting duct by uric acid crystals. The urine pH is lowest in these nephron segments, facilitating urate precipitation. Local reaction by tubular cells is also implicated.
- Laboratory studies suggest that primary protection is not achieved by alkalinizing the urine but by maintaining a high urine flow rate. Equivalent protection is provided by water-induced or loop diuretic-induced diuresis.
- Pre-treatment of patients with allopurinol and saline-loading for several days minimizes the incidence of ARF in clinical practice.

Radiocontrast-induced ARF

- This is more frequent in patients of advanced age, and in those with CRF, myeloma or diabetes mellitus. It is more likely to occur in these patients if there is ECF depletion, poor left ventricular function and use of high doses of contrast (>125 ml).

- Most ARF is mild, with a non-oliguric transient rise of plasma creatinine concentration in patients with normal initial renal function. Characteristically there is a low urinary sodium concentration.
- Intense vacuolization of proximal tubular cells is a non-specific feature of renal biopsy. Functional studies suggest that the principal damage is to the MTALH.
- Non-ionic contrast agents cause fewer allergic reactions and cardiovascular reactions: ARF is less common, but only in high risk patients. Adequate hydration prior to the procedure minimizes the incidence of ARF. No additional protection is provided by other interventions. The principal risk factor is pre-existing CRF.

Further reading

Ratcliffe P. Pathophysiology of acute renal failure. In: Cameron JS, Davison AM, Grünfeld J-P, Kerr D, Ritz E (eds) *Oxford Textbook of Clinical Nephrology*. Oxford: Oxford University Press, 1992; 982–1005.

Rudnick MR, Berns JS, Cohen RM, Goldfarb S. Contrast media-associated nephrotoxicity. *Current Opinion in Nephrology and Hypertension,* 1996; **5**: 127–33.

Related topics of interest

ACUTE RENAL FAILURE: GENERAL APPROACH

Acute renal failure (ARF) is a not uncommon accompaniment of illness. It is associated with a high mortality rate. Recovery of renal function is the usual outcome if the patient survives the effects of the associated illness.

Epidemiology

- The annual incidence of ARF in a community has been estimated at 850–900 cases per million population (pmp). Not all cases are severe. Many resolve without specific therapy.
- More severe ARF ([creatinine] >500 µmol/l), during which the patient may die or require renal replacement therapy, has an incidence of $c.140$ cases pmp per annum. Incidence increases with increasing age. Annual incidence is greater than 750 cases pmp in patients older than 80 years.
- Excluding patients who die rapidly of associated conditions (e.g. elderly patients with severe ARF in the context of cardiogenic shock), the annual incidence of severe ARF which will require specific therapy is probably 50–100 cases pmp.
- About 33% of cases of severe ARF are due to obstruction, 10–15% to surgical and cardio-vascular causes, and about 10% to sepsis and ECF volume depletion.
- ARF is more common (70%) in male patients. Even when cases of obstructive prostatic disease are excluded, males still constitute about 66% of cases.
- Patient survival following ARF is about 50% at 3 months and 33% at 2 years. Death is usually due to associated or co-morbid conditions.
- Mild ARF ([creatinine] >150 µmol/l) occurs in 10% of all hospitalized patients, 20% of trauma patients, 10% of elective and 50% of emergency aortic surgery patients. More severe ARF ([creatinine] >350 µmol/l) occurs in 2%, 5%, 15% and 25%, respectively, of the above groups.

Definitions

- ARF is a decline in renal function occurring over hours or days.

- It may occur from a normal or abnormal baseline level of function.
- It may be oliguric (urine volume <500 ml/day) or non-oliguric.
- It is usually associated with rising plasma urea and creatinine concentrations.
- Glomerular and tubular function are both deranged. Accumulation of nitrogenous wastes and H^+ ions occurs. There is inability to regulate water and electrolyte balance. Endocrine function derangements do not usually cause immediate clinical problems.
- Oliguria due to salt and water retention (heart failure, nephrotic syndrome) or as a physiological response to mild ECF volume depletion or stress (e.g. surgery) is not ARF. Oliguria due to urinary retention is not ARF.
- Patients with advanced CRF or ESRF occasionally present as uraemic emergencies. These cases behave differently to ARF cases as their underlying pathology is different.

Conceptual framework

- ARF is always due to a nephrotoxic insult (or, more usually, insults) which almost always occurs in the setting of pre-existing risk factors. Insults may be ischaemic, immunological, toxic or mechanical. Insults are usually identifiable, frequently predictable and often avoidable.
- Risk factors pre-disposing to ARF in response to insults are usually identifiable and can sometimes be modified.
- ARF is uncommon as an isolated illness arising in the community but common as one of a number of illnesses in a hospitalized patient.
- In ARF, patient death is common (*c.* 50%) but permanent renal failure is uncommon (*c.* 5%). Most cases of ARF will recover, provided the patient survives the associated illness.

Insults

- Ischaemic insults include haemorrhage, burns, vomiting, diarrhoea or anything that interferes with ECF volume status. Cardiovascular derangements such as myocardial infarction, cardiac dysrythmias, left ventricular dysfunction, sepsis and shock are also ischaemic insults, as are, changes in intra-renal haemodynamics due to NSAIDs. Such insults could be described as 'pre-renal'.

- Immunological insults may be autoimmune or allergic. Idiopathic glomerulonephritis is an unusual cause of ARF. However, systemic ill-nesses such as Wegener's granulomatosis, SLE and anti-GBM disease frequently present as ARF. Allergic interstitial nephritis, due to drug therapy, and cholesterol embolization are other common immunological insults. Such insults could be described as 'renal'.

- Toxic insults such as aminoglycosides, foscarnet, paraquat and radiocontrast agents could also be described as 'renal' insults.

- Obvious mechanical insults include intrinsic and extrinsic obstruction to the ureter, as might happen with a ureteric calculus and a pelvic tumour respectively. As they evolve, most cases of ARF will include a degree of tubular ob-struction. These could be described as 'post-renal' insults.

- It is usual for a few of these insults to occur simultaneously. Vigilance in patient care, especially with regard to fluid balance, drug pre-scription and treatment of sepsis is important in identifying and avoiding the principal causes of ARF.

Risk factors

- With increasing age, GFR frequently declines even in 'healthy normals'. Increased co-prevalence of other risk factors place the elderly at high risk for ARF. They also have less renal and cardiac reserve in the face of ECF depletion, sepsis or surgery.

- Existing CRF increases the risk of ARF, as does long-standing cardiac and hepatic failure. Diffuse vascular disease, with the possibility of renal artery stenosis, is a frequent risk factor.

- Dementia and immobility interfere with patients' ability to regulate their own fluid balance, as do high-output fistulae or chronic diarrhoeal conditions.

- Continuing 'usual medications' in ill, hospitalized patients may predispose them to ARF, especially if NSAIDs, ACEIs and diuretics are amongst the list. All prescriptions must be justified continuously.

Assessment and investigations

- Identification of pre-existing risk factors and of all nephrotoxic insults is most important. Clinical assessment of the patient with particular focus on ECF volume status, cardiovascular function and presence of sepsis must be immediate and comprehensive. Central access to measure right- or left-sided cardiac filling pressures may be neccessary to achieve this.
- Plasma biochemistry to identify urea, creatinine, sodium, potassium, bicarbonate and calcium levels. Full blood count and clotting screen.
- Dipstick urinalysis to seek haematuria and proteinuria, supplemented, if necessary, by urine microscopy.
- Culture of blood, urine and other appropriate fluids depending on circumstances.
- Tests involving assessment of plasma:urinary sodium and osmolality ratios are almost impossible to interpret and should not be done.
- CXR to seek the presence of pulmonary oedema or haemorrhage.
- ECG to seek evidence of cardiac dysfunction or hyperkalaemia. Echocardiography to exclude pericardial effusion and tamponade, if suspected.
- Ultrasonography to exclude obstruction and assess renal size is mandatory. Selective renal arteriography or isotope studies may be indicated if a vascular catastrophe is suspected, but this is not without hazard to renal function. Anterograde or retrograde uretero-pyelography may be indicated in cases of obstruction. There is practically no indication for IVU.
- ANCA, ANF or anti-GBM assay if clinically indicated.

- Renal biopsy is indicated only if drug-induced AIN, glomerulonephritis, vasculitis, scleroderma renal crisis or other 'medical condition' is suspected. May also be indicated if apparently 'straightforward ATN' is slow to recover.

Management

- Most management is supportive, with emphasis on removing ongoing nephrotoxic insults, maintaining fluid balance, treating sepsis, minimizing electrolyte and metabolic derangements and maintaining adequate caloric and protein nutrition. RRT can be avoided in many cases by this approach.
- All unnecessary and toxic medications should be discontinued. Patients with ECF volume depletion should have this corrected with appropriate fluid therapy. Cardiac dysrythmias should be treated, pericardial effusions drained, sepsis treated by antibiotics and surgical drainage, urinary tract obstructions relieved perurethrally or percutaneously and specific therapy given to patients with vasculitis, HUS/TTP or other conditions.
- Patients with multi-organ failure due to trauma, sepsis or other major illness should be managed in the ITU environment with optimization of circulatory function and control of oxygenation.
- If it is felt that the patient can be managed conservatively, then fastidious restriction of fluids and electrolytes should be imposed. This may be easier with non-oliguric ARF. However, if nutrition is compromised because of this, RRT should be used. Discussion with the local renal service may be helpful.
- RRT is indicated if patients are severely compromised by metabolic, electrolyte or fluid imbalance. If it is evident that these problems will worsen on conservative management, RRT should be started in anticipation of the problem.
- During the recovery phase, a marked diuresis is often seen. Maintaining ECF volume status and electrolyte levels will require frequent review and adjustment of therapy.

Use of diuretics

- Mannitol and loop diuretics have theoretically attractive functions in ARF. By maintaining diuresis they wash out cellular debris, prevent tubular obstruction, prevent pre-glomerular vasoconstriction and inhibit glomerulotubular feedback. Mannitol may scavenge free radicals and minimize post-ischaemic swelling. These findings have mainly been seen in experimental models or following renal transplantation.

- Due to the heterogeneity of insults and risk factors in clinical disease, it is unclear if diuretics are of benefit. Most studies showing benefit paid more fastidious attention to ECF volume status than might occur in clinical practice and began the diuretics before, or at the point of, insult. In clinical practice, diuretics may convert oliguric to non-oliguric ARF, which may help management of fluid balance, but there is little to suggest any other benefit.

- In multi-organ failure, some studies indicate that low-dose frusemide may be of benefit in preventing or ameliorating ARF if given to patients with an optimal left-ventricular filling pressure, adequate cardiac output and adequate mean arterial pressure. In theory it acts to protect MTALH from ischaemia by inhibiting its local $Na^+-K^+-2Cl^-$ co-transporter pump. Such patients generally have a Swan–Ganz catheter *in situ*, are on assisted ventilation, dobutamine, angiotensin and/or noradrenaline so it is difficult to extrapolate to other clinical scenarios.

Low-dose dopamine

- This is the traditional but contentious adjunct to the general care of patients with established ARF. There is some evidence, mainly from patients with normal renal function, that sub-inotropic doses may increase renal blood flow. It is a natriuretic agent and may convert patients from oliguric to non-oliguric ARF. There is little evidence that it improves the GFR in a clinical setting.

- It may be harmful in sepsis because of splanchnic vasodilatation and interference with carotid baro-receptor function.
- It may be indirectly beneficial by 'upgrading care' and requiring central access to be established, with transfer of the patient to a higher dependency care unit.

Further reading

Denton MD, Chertow GM, Brady HR. 'Renal-dose' dopamine for the treatment of acute renal failure: Scientific rationale, experimental studies and clinical trials. *Kidney International* 1996, **49**: 4–14.

Kleinknecht D. Management of acute renal failure. In: Cameron JS, Davison AM, Grünfeld J-P, Kerr D, Ritz E (eds) *Oxford Textbook of Clinical Nephrology.* Oxford: Oxford University Press, 1992; 1015–26.

Rainford DJ, Stevens PE. The investigative approach to the patient with acute renal failure. In: Cameron JS, Davison AM, Grünfeld J-P, Kerr D, Ritz E (eds)*Oxford Textbook of Clinical Nephrology.* Oxford: Oxford University Press, 1992; 969–82.

Related topics of interest

Acute renal failure: acute tubular necrosis and selected syndromes (p. 7)
Drug induced renal disease (p. 57)
Haemolytic uraemic syndrome and thrombotic thrombocytopenic purpura (p. 98)
Rapidly progressive glomerulonephritis (p. 149)
Renal biopsy (p. 163)

ANALGESIC NEPHROPATHY

Analgesic nephropathy is a significant cause of endstage renal failure (ESRF) in a number of countries. Protracted regular consumption of large doses of compound analgesic agents leads to a chronic interstitial nephropathy.

Aetiology

- Regional variations in prevalence parallel variations in patterns of analgesic use. There is a marked association with daily usage for more than 5 years of compound antipyretic–analgesic preparations. Phenacetin and aspirin are frequently found in such combinations, which often have added codeine or caffeine ('2+1' agents).
- It is unusual with long-term consumption of paracetamol, aspirin or NSAIDs as single-agent preparations.
- Increasing analgesic concentrations down the medullary concentration gradient decrease local reducing substances, with consequent increases in reactive intermediary metabolites. This leads to tubulointerstitial changes, beginning at the papilla.
- Cortical lesions follow, from decreased renal plasma flow in response to papillary and tubulointerstitial damage. Papillary necrosis may occur, especially in the setting of ECF depletion.

Prevalence

- Impaired urinary concentrating ability is found in up to 25% of patients with a heavy consumption of compound analgesic preparations for over 10 years. Raised plasma creatinine concentration is found in 6–7% of such patients.
- It is especially prevalent in Australia, Germany, Switzerland, Sweden, Austria and Belgium, accounting for up to 30% of cases of ESRF in certain regions.
- More common in women, with a peak incidence in the sixth decade.

Problems

- Asymptomatic or with non-specific symptoms in early stages.

- Impaired urinary concentrating ability is the earliest clinical sign, which may present as polyuria or ECF volume depletion.
- Distal hypokalaemic RTA occurs in 15% of patients.
- CRF progressing to ESRF.
- Papillary necrosis may present as haematuria and loin pain or (less commonly) with ureteric obstruction.
- Urothelial malignancy occurs in up to 10% of cases. The increased risk is more marked for renal pelvic cancer than for renal cell carcinoma. Loin pain and haematuria are suggestive but not specific symptoms.

Investigations

- A careful history of the pattern, frequency, duration and nature of analgesic consumption should be taken. Patients may deny or conceal these details. Urine may be screened for the presence of analgesic metabolites.
- Sterile pyuria is a highly specific finding.
- Renal ultrasound scanning and computed tomography are the imaging techniques of greatest sensitivity and specificity. The finding of a bilateral decrease in renal size, with both kidneys having irregular contours, is characteristic. Additional specific findings include intra-renal ring calcification and papillary necrosis.
- Impaired urinary concentrating ability may be detected in response to water deprivation. This is more marked with renal failure.
- An inability to achieve maximum urinary acidification in response to acid-loading reveals the presence of a distal renal tubular acidosis.
- Haematuria, especially if macroscopic, raises the possibility of acute papillary necrosis or urothelial malignancy. Appropriate investigations include urine cytology, radiological studies and endoscopic urological examination of the renal tract.
- Features of CRF will be found but are not specific to this condition.

Management	• Identification of the cause and immediate cessation of analgesic consumption may halt the progression of renal impairment and possibly allow some recovery of function.
	• Excessive ECF volume depletion should be avoided. This will further impair renal plasma flow and possibly precipitate papillary necrosis. Excessive use (or concomitant abuse) of diuretics must be avoided.
	• Urinary infection should be treated aggressively.
	• Conservative management of CRF.
	• ESRF should be treated by dialysis and/or transplantation.
	• Long-term surveillance for the development of urothelial malignancy is important, even after cessation of analgesic consumption and especially after transplantation.
Differential diagnosis	• Analgesic nephropathy needs to be distinguished from other causes of chronic interstitial nephropathy and renal papillary necrosis such as lead nephropathy, sickle-cell disease, reflux nephropathy and Balkan nephropathy.

Further reading

Heinrich WL. Analgesic nephropathy. *American Journal of Medical Science,* 1988; **295**: 561–8.

Related topics of interest

ASSESSMENT OF THE PATIENT WITH RENAL DISEASE

Renal diseases vary from asymptomatic abnormalities of questionable clinical significance to rapidly progressive and life-threatening diseases. Many of the diseases that ultimately cause renal failure are initially asymptomatic.

Presenting features of renal disease

Nephrotic syndrome

Nephrotic syndrome presents with the triad of oedema, hypoalbuminaemia and proteinuria (>3 g/24 h). Facial oedema, most marked in the morning, is characteristic, particularly in children. Pulmonary oedema may occur at very low serum albumin levels. Causes include minimal change disease, membranous glomerulonephritis and most other types of glomerular disease. Renal biopsy is required for an accurate diagnosis, although children with a characteristic presentation are assumed to have minimal change disease.

Nephritic syndrome

This is defined as the combination of oliguric renal failure, haematuria and proteinuria, and hypertension, with or without oedema. This may occur in rapidly progressive glomerulonephritis and in a number of other glomerular diseases, such as post-streptococcal glomerulonephritis and haemolytic uraemic syndrome.

Hypertension

High blood pressure, particularly if there is no family history of essential hypertension, may be the first sign of renal artery stenosis or intrinsic renal disease.

Chronic renal failure

Symptoms of chronic renal failure are often non-specific and include malaise, tiredness, anorexia, nausea and vomiting, itching, restless legs and insomnia. Thirst, polyuria and nocturia may occur.

Renal bone disease	Occasionally the presenting feature of renal disease is bone pain and proximal muscle weakness due to renal bone disease.
Incidental findings	Renal disease is often first detected on routine screening, either on urinalysis (haematuria and/or proteinuria); full blood count (normochromic normocytic anaemia); or biochemical screening (raised urea and creatinine).

History

General	Any of the symptoms listed above should alert one to the possibility of renal disease. Any history of renal disease or urological surgery in the past is relevant. Pregnancy-induced hypertension or pre-eclampsia may, in retrospect, be clues to pre-existing renal disease. Symptoms of bladder outflow obstruction should be enquired about.
Occupation	Exposure to organic solvents may increase the risk of glomerulonephritis. Heavy metals, including cadmium and lead, are nephrotoxic.
Smoking	Smokers with diabetes are more likely to develop diabetic nephropathy than otherwise similar non-smoking diabetics. Smoking also increases the risk of subsequent non-diabetic renal disease, probably by causing atherosclerosis of the renal arteries and intrarenal vascular disease.
Alcohol	Contrary to popular myth, alcohol use does not cause renal disease.
Family history	Familial renal diseases include polycystic renal disease, medullary cystic disease, and Alport's syndrome. Often these diseases may not have been diagnosed accurately in the past, so any family history of renal disease or renal failure should be taken seriously. Reflux nephropathy also has a strong familial component.

Surgical history	A history of surgery to the urinary tract should raise the possibility of recurrent obstruction or of infection. Renal stones may recur and cause obstruction. Recurrent stone formation raises the possibility of primary hyperoxaluria. Bowel resection, as for Crohn's, or small bowel bypass surgery for obesity, may also cause recurrent oxalate stones. Ileostomy patients are prone to recurrent hypovolaemia and urate stones.
Drugs	Drugs that can cause renal disease include analgesics, non-steroidal anti-inflammatory drugs, gold, penicillamine, aminoglycosides and *cis-* platinum.

Physical examination

General	Non-specific signs include white nails, pallor, and increased skin pigmentation. Assessment of fluid balance is very important and includes assessment of oedema, skin turgor, jugular venous pressure and blood pressure in the lying and standing positions.
Skin	Vasculitic rashes are usually caused by small-vessel vasculitis, which causes skin haemorrhage and necrosis. Nodular prurigo and widespread scratch marks can cause diagnostic confusion. Livedo reticularis may occur in SLE, the antiphospholipid syndrome and in cholesterol embolism.
Joints	Patients with rheumatoid arthritis are at risk of renal disease either as a direct result of rheumatoid vasculitis or as a result of drug therapy. Gout is relatively common in patients with renal disease but is not a cause of renal disease *per se*.
Urine	Urinalysis is part of the examination of every patient.

Blood tests

Urea	Urea is a product of amino-acid catabolism in the liver and is excreted by a combination of glomerular filtration and tubular secretion in the kidneys. Serum

urea concentration reflects the balance between production and removal. Production is increased by steroids, catabolic stress and gastrointestinal bleeding, and is decreased by liver disease. Removal is decreased by congestive cardiac failure, hypovolaemia and diuretic treatment. By itself, therefore, urea concentration is not a good guide to renal excretory function.

Creatinine

Creatinine is produced at a constant rate from muscle, and unless there is acute muscle damage, endogenous creatinine production is directly related to muscle mass. Apart from a small amount of tubular secretion, creatinine is eliminated by glomerular filtration. Serum creatinine concentration is determined by the following relationship:

[creatinine] = production rate/clearance rate.

Because production rate is constant (and equal to excretion rate), this means that serum creatinine is inversely related to clearance.

In a subject of average build, serum creatinine does not rise outside the normal range until clearance is 50% normal. In subjects with low muscle mass (for instance, elderly females), serum creatinine may not become abnormal until clearance is 30% normal. Serum creatinine is therefore a good marker for significant renal impairment but not for early renal impairment.

Creatinine clearance

Creatinine clearance is a readily available way of estimating glomerular filtration rate and is calculated by dividing the 24 h creatinine production rate by the serum creatinine concentration. The major problems are in ensuring a complete and accurate 24 h collection, particularly in patients with impaired bladder emptying. Tubular secretion of creatinine contributes significantly to creatinine clearance in patients with low glomerular filtration rates, and can be inhibited by cimetidine and trimethaprim.

Creatinine clearance may be estimated from age, gender, weight and serum creatinine by the Cockcroft and Gault formula:

$$\text{estimated clearance} = \{(140 - \text{age}[y]) \times \text{weight}[kg]/\text{creatinine}[\mu mol/l]\} \times 1.23[\text{male}] \text{ or } 1.04[\text{female}].$$

Isotopic clearance Accurate measurement of glomerular filtration rate is seldom required except for research purposes. If necessary, clearance of radiolabelled inulin, EDTA, or iothalamate can be measured by taking repeated blood samples after a bolus injection. The normal glomerular filtration rate is approximately 125 ml/min/1.73 m^2 body surface area, declining by around 10 ml/min/m^2/decade after the age of 40.

Further reading

Levey AS. Clinical evaluation of renal function. In: Greenberg A (ed.) *Primer on Renal Diseases*. London: Academic Press, 1994; 17–23.

Related topics of interest

Acute renal failure: general approach (p. 7)
Glomerulonephritis: general approach (p. 81)
Imaging of the urinary tract (p. 110)
Renal biopsy (p. 163)
Urinalysis and urine microscopy (p. 215)

AUTOSOMAL DOMINANT POLYCYSTIC KIDNEY DISEASE

Autosomal dominant polycystic kidney disease (ADPKD) is a common disorder with a worldwide prevalence of 1 in 500 to 1 in 1000. It is an important cause of hypertension in younger patients and causes progressive chronic renal failure (CRF), frequently leading to endstage renal failure (ESRF). Eight to ten per cent of all dialysis patients have ADPKD. It should not be confused with acquired cystic kidney disease which occurs in patients with long-standing renal failure and is not familial.

Problems

- Hypertension.
- CRF and ESRF.
- Haematuria.
- Urinary tract infection.
- Loin pain.
- Subarachnoid haemorrhage.
- Genetic counselling.

Pathophysiology

- Multiple cysts, lined by tubular-type cells, develop in the cortex and medulla of both kidneys. These contain uriniferous fluid, altered blood or pyogenic secretions. Intervening areas of the kidney show nephrosclerosis and chronic interstitial nephropathy. A variety of abnormalities of cell proliferation and matrix production have been demonstrated.
- Cysts also develop in the liver (30–50% of patients); hepatocellular damage is rare, but obstruction of major bile ducts or the portal venous system can lead to jaundice or portal hypertension. Cysts also occur in other organs, including the pancreas, spleen, ovary and testis. Colonic diverticulosis is more common than in the general population.
- Heart valve abnormalities, principally mitral valve prolapse (25% of patients), are more frequent than in the general population.
- Subarachnoid haemorrhage (SAH), associated with intracerebral berry aneurysms, occurs in approximately 10% of patients. The prevalence of aneurysms in asymptomatic patients is

unknown but they may be more common in affected relatives of patients who have had SAH.

Genetics

- Gene linkage is seen in 90–95% of affected families, with markers on chromosome 16 (PKD1 families). Recently, the gene itself has been identified. The existence of other affected families without this genotype (non-PKD1) suggests that more than one gene defect may produce the phenotype.
- Inheritance shows autosomal dominance. Onset of symptoms may be earlier if the disease is inherited from the mother. The rate of progression of CRF shows less variability within families than between families.
- A positive family history is obtained in the majority of cases. Its absence suggests unsuspected non-paternity or spontaneous mutation.

Clinical features

- ADPKD does not usually become symptomatic until the third or fourth decades of life and is subsequently progressive.

1. Hypertension. This occurs in 25% of children and young adults and in 65% of adults. Initially it may reflect an activated renin–angiotensin system due to intra-renal ischaemia. As CRF develops, the contribution of salt and water retention to hypertension becomes more marked.

2. Haematuria. Occurs in over 50% of patients and may be microscopic or macroscopic (often causing severe alarm to the patient). It is usually felt to represent rupture of a cyst into the renal pelvis.

3. Loin pain. Pain may be severe and reflect cyst rupture, haemorrhage or infection within a cyst, or urolithiasis (10% of ADPKD patients pass renal stones).

4. Urinary tract infection. UTI may not be more frequent in these patients but is often difficult to eradicate.

5. *An abdominal mass.* A mass may be found at incidental examination, or be noticed by the patient.

6. *CRF or ESRF.* CRF or even ESRF may be the first manifestation.

7. *Renal carcinoma.* This is probably not more frequent in ADPKD than in the normal population.

8. *Screening.* Screening of relatives of affected probands now detects an increasing proportion of cases. At the time of diagnosis 30–40% of affected relatives will already have unsuspected complications. Completely asymptomatic patients are also detected by screening.

Progression

This disease progresses throughout life. CRF will often progress at a similar rate to that experienced by other affected family members. Not all patients progress to ESRF (50–60%). Studies suggest that the median age for development of ESRF for PKD1 families is around 56 years, and 68 years for non-PKD1 families. Rigorous control of hypertension is important in attenuating the rate of progression.

Clinical assessment

- Family history is of paramount importance.
- Bimanual palpation of the abdomen will detect bilaterally enlarged kidneys, with an irregular surface, in the majority of cases. Hepatomegaly may also be detected.
- Measurement of blood pressure and evaluation of other clinical evidence of hypertensive end-organ damage.
- Clinical features of CRF may be detected. These may be relatively non-specific. Anaemia is less frequently seen in this condition than in other causes of CRF.

Investigations

- Renal function tests to evaluate the degree of CRF.
- Urine microscopy and culture to detect haematuria or urinary tract infection.

- Ultrasound (USS) examination of the abdomen is extremely sensitive and specific in the diagnosis of APKD in patients aged over 30 years. Multiple cysts are seen in both kidneys. Hepatic and pancreatic cysts may also be visualized. In younger patients there is an increased incidence of false negative examinations when compared with gene linkage analysis. Absence of cysts on USS cannot completely exclude subsequent expression of the ADPKD phenotype in patients under 30 years and especially in those under 10 years (36% false negative rate).
- Computed tomography (CT) is more sensitive than USS. The increased cost and radiation exposure of this technique militates against its use in asymptomatic individuals.
- Intravenous urography (IVU) is not now indicated if either of the above techniques is available.
- Cerebral arteriography is not routinely advised unless an SAH has occurred. Less invasive techniques such as magnetic resonance imaging are currently under evaluation in this context.
- Gene linkage analysis is now available, although not on a routine basis. It may be helpful in screening younger asymptomatic relatives of probands in PKD1 families, particularly if advice regarding conception is sought.

Management

- Hypertension should be controlled by correcting salt and water retention and by antihypertensive agents. Because of the postulated role of an activated renin–angiotensin system it is rational to incorporate an ACE inhibitor in the regime, if this does not compromise renal function.
- CRF should be managed conservatively as for any cause and as detailed in the related section of this book.
- ESRF should be treated by dialysis and, when appropriate, transplantation. Occasionally, very large kidneys militate against the use of peritoneal dialysis and uninephrectomy may be

necessary prior to transplantation. Combined liver and kidney transplants have been performed.
- Urinary tract infections may not respond well to conventional therapeutic regimes. Water-soluble and cationic antibiotics penetrate cysts poorly. Quinolones may thus be more efficacious than aminoglycoside or β-lactam antibiotics. Drainage may be necessary in resistant cases.
- Haematuria rarely requires specific treatment.
- Loin pain is treated by analgesic agents. Surgical puncture of cysts (Rovsing's procedure) is currently under evaluation for this indication.

Further reading

Pirson Y, Grünfeld J-P. Autosomal-dominant polycystic kidney disease. In: Cameron S, Davison AM, Grünfeld J-P, Kerr D, Ritz E (eds) *Oxford Textbook of Clinical Nephrology*. Oxford: Oxford University Press, 1992; 2171–87.

Related topics of interest

CHRONIC RENAL FAILURE

Significant loss of renal excretory function is relatively common: a serum creatinine of above 300 µmol/l is found in 450 pmp of the population and above 500 µmol/l in 132 per million. Mild to moderate chronic renal failure results in few symptoms and may remain undetected until complications of renal failure occur.

Presenting features

1. Symptoms. These include loss of appetite, nausea and vomiting; itching; polyuria and nocturia; restless legs; insomnia; and symptoms of anaemia. These do not usually become prominent until glomerular filtration rate is 15% of normal. Severe renal failure causes mental obtundation, myoclonic twitching, and eventual coma.

2. Signs. There are no specific physical signs of uraemia. Poor nutrition or hypoalbuminaemia may cause leuconychia. Itching may result in scratch marks. Increased skin pigmentation can occur. Glove and stocking peripheral neuropathy may occur but its presence before endstage renal failure should raise the possibility of an alternative cause.

Urinalysis may reveal proteinuria and/or haematuria, depending on the underlying cause.

3. Incidental finding. Often chronic renal failure is detected as part of a 'routine' biochemical screen in patients with no symptoms. It is seldom justified to ignore a raised serum creatinine level, as it indicates that 50% of renal function has already been lost, and further progression may occur unless the cause is identified and treated.

Investigation

Chronic renal failure is usually confirmed by measurement of serum creatinine or creatinine clearance. Sometimes the cause is known or obvious from the history (including drug history) and examination, but frequently no such clues are present.

1. Acute or chronic? If there is no history of uraemic symptoms to give clues to the duration of disease, the most reliable indicator of chronicity is renal size, usually measured as renal length on ultrasound. Decreased renal size and increased renal echogenicity indicate chronic disease, although some causes of chronic renal failure may be associated with normal-sized kidneys (e.g. diabetes, amyloidosis). The presence of renal bone disease and anaemia also suggests chronicity, although anaemia may appear within days of acute renal failure, depending on the cause.

2. Underlying cause. Glomerulonephritis may be suggested by urinalysis and (sometimes) by autoantibody tests and complement assays, and confirmed by biopsy. In older patients urine and serum electrophoresis for myeloma should be performed. Intravenous urography (IVU) is required for diagnosis of reflux nephropathy and analgesic nephropathy. Hydronephrosis on ultrasound or IVU suggests obstruction. Polycystic disease is best demonstrated with ultrasound.

Complications

- Anaemia.
- Hypertension.
- Left ventricular hypertrophy.
- Increased cardiovascular mortality.
- Hypertriglyceridaemia.
- Impaired drug elimination.
- Bone disease, vascular and extra-articular calcification.
- Pericarditis (late).
- Neuropathy (late).

Progression

Progressive renal damage may continue to occur independently of the initiating disease, for instance in reflux nephropathy or after an episode of obstructive nephropathy or accelerated hypertension. This phenomenon is thought to be due to maladaptive 'compensatory' changes (hypertrophy and hyperfiltration) in surviving nephrons and is more likely the more renal mass has been lost in the initial insult. Proteinuria and hypertension are common concomitants of this so-called 'remnant nephropathy'. In addition, the initiating disease may continue to cause renal damage, as in some forms of glomerulonephritis, polycystic disease, and diabetic nephropathy.

Management

1. Underlying disease. Specific treatments are available for some forms of glomerulonephritis.

2. Hypertension. This should be carefully controlled. In diabetic nephropathy, and probably in other proteinuric renal diseases, ACE inhibitors appear to be more effective at slowing progression than equipotent doses of other antihypertensives; however, they cause renal failure in patients with renal artery stenosis and may cause or exacerbate hyperkalaemia. Loop diuretics are useful in controlling hypertension due to volume overload and potentiate the effects of ACE inhibitors.

3. Hyperparathyroidism. This should be searched for and controlled.

4. Anaemia. This can be treated with erythropoietin if symptoms are severe. Concern that this might accelerate progression has not yet proved to be justified.

5. Acidosis. Acidosis should be corrected to avert bone disease and muscle wasting.

6. Hyperlipidaemia. In view of the high relative risk of cardiovascular disease in renal failure it seems sensible to detect and treat hyperlipidaemia. Experimental studies suggest that correction of hypercholesterolaemia may retard progression, but this has not yet been demonstrated in humans.

7. Avoidance of further insults. Non-steroidal anti-inflammatory drugs, tetracyclines, aminoglycosides and other nephrotoxic agents should be avoided.

Acute hypovolaemia may precipitate acute or chronic renal failure, particularly in patients on ACE inhibitors; causes include diuretics and gastroenteritis.

8. *Drug doses.* These should be adjusted to avoid accumulation if they are renally cleared. This is particularly important for hypoglycaemic agents and allopurinol.

9. *Preparation for endstage renal failure.* This should include counselling on the future need for dialysis and/or transplantation and advance planning for the dialysis modality most suitable for the individual patient. If haemodialysis is planned, an arteriovenous fistula should be created at least 3 months before it is likely to be needed. Reasonable predictions on the timing of endstage renal failure can be made from graphical plotting of 1/creatinine against time. Late referral for dialysis is associated with increased morbidity and mortality.

Further reading

de Zeeuw D, Apperloo AJ, de Jong P. Management of chronic renal failure. *Current Opinion in Nephrology and Hypertension*, 1992; **1**: 116–23.
Jacobson HR. Chronic renal failure: pathophysiology. *Lancet*, 1991; **338**: 419–23.
Klahr S. Chronic renal failure: management. *Lancet*, 1991; **338**: 423–7.

Related topics of interest

COMPLICATIONS OF THE NEPHROTIC SYNDROME

Renal vein thrombosis

Renal vein thrombosis is an important cause of renal impairment in patients with nephrotic syndrome, and is frequently undiagnosed. It may also occur as a complication of renal transplantation and in renal malignancy.

Causes

1. Membranous nephropathy. This appears to have a particular predilection for causing renal vein thrombosis: the reason for this association is unknown.

2. Lupus nephritis. This is also associated with renal vein thrombosis, whether or not in association with membranous glomerulonephritis. Anti-cardiolipin antibodies may confer an increased risk, but this is uncertain.

3. Amyloidosis. This is frequently associated with thrombosis of small intrarenal veins, which may subsequently propagate to involve the main renal vein.

4. Any other form of glomerulonephritis causing nephrotic syndrome may also be complicated by thrombosis.

Clinical features

Renal vein thrombosis may be completely asymptomatic, or may cause:

- Loin pain.
- Haematuria.
- Renal swelling.
- Acute renal failure or acute on chronic renal failure with oliguria.

Extension to the vena cava may cause:

- Bilateral leg swelling.
- Pulmonary emboli.

The frequency of pulmonary emboli in renal thrombosis is over 30%. Massive or fatal pulmonary embolism is surprisingly rare.

Frequency

Because diagnosis requires complicated tests, the true frequency is unknown. Renal vein thrombosis can be found in up to 50% of patients with membranous nephropathy and nephrotic syndrome, but is symptomatic in only 5–15%. Asymptomatic abnormalities on ventilation perfusion scanning may be found in over 10% of adult nephrotic patients, but some cases of pulmonary emboli may derive from deep venous thrombosis in the leg veins, which also occurs more frequently in nephrotic patients.

Pathogenesis

- Immobility.
- Volume contraction as a result of hypo-albuminaemia and diuretics, causing increased whole blood viscosity.
- Increased plasma fibrinogen, causing increased plasma viscosity.
- Urinary loss of anticoagulant or regulatory proteins in excess of procoagulant proteins.
- Increased platelet adhesiveness (?)

Natural history

Untreated, symptomatic renal vein thrombosis causes progressive and irreversible renal failure, as well as extension into the inferior vena cava and systemic embolism. How frequently this occurs in asymptomatic cases is uncertain.

Diagnosis

The diagnosis should be suspected in a predisposed patient who develops haematuria, acute renal failure, or flank pain, particularly if this occurs in the context of acute volume depletion. It is not considered justified to investigate asymptomatic patients.

1. Cross-linked fibrin degradation products. Elevated levels have been shown to be sensitive for detection of deep venous thrombosis and pulmonary embolism, but have not been investigated in renal vein thrombosis.

2. *Ultrasound.* The kidneys appear swollen, with loss of the normal corticomedullary differentiation. On Duplex scanning, decreased or absent flow may be seen in the renal veins, but these are sometimes hard to image: normal flow can help to exclude the diagnosis but failure to demonstrate flow is unhelpful. Arterial flow patterns show evidence of greatly increased resistance to flow, with reversal in diastole.

3. *Venography.* This is invasive and requires injection of contrast into the renal veins against the direction of flow after selective catheterization. Renal vein thrombosis causes filling defects (although artefacts are common) and decreased washout.

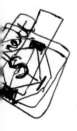

4. *Arteriography.* The renal veins should be demonstrated clearly on the venous phase.

5. *Magnetic resonance angiography.* This technique is under evaluation and may become the modality of choice in the future.

6. *Renal biopsy.* This may show characteristic appearances, with margination of neutrophils and vascular congestion.

Management

Unless there are strong contraindications, all patients should be fully anticoagulated. Warfarin is bound to albumin, so changes in serum albumin may necessitate adjustment in dose. The duration for which anticoagulation is required is uncertain, but it would be rational to continue anticoagulation until the nephrotic syndrome has resolved.

Thrombolysis has been used in patients with acute renal failure and pulmonary emboli, but experience is limited.

Hypercholesterolaemia

A greatly raised total cholesterol is nearly always seen in nephrotic patients. Several long-term studies have demonstrated an increased risk of death from coronary artery disease in patients with a history of nephrotic syndrome, suggesting that atherogenesis is accelerated by secondary hypercholesterolaemia. Whether hypercholesterolaemia contributes to progression of renal disease remains uncertain, although there is strong suggestive evidence that it does.

Pathogenesis	Increased hepatic cholesterol synthesis appears to be 'switched on' by decreased plasma oncotic pressure: the mechanism is uncertain.
Treatment	The results of dietary treatment are often disappointing. HMG CoA–reductase inhibitors ('statins') are effective and probably the drugs of choice. Drug treatment should be actively considered, particularly in patients in whom the chances of remission are slight.

Infection

Infection was the predominant cause of death in minimal change disease until steroid treatment was introduced, and remains an important cause of morbidity and mortality.

Presentation	*1. Spontaneous bacterial peritonitis.* Occurs particularly in nephrotic children and may be rapidly progressive. This is frequently due to Pneumococcus.
	2. Cellulitis. This is a frequent problem in adults.
Pathogenesis	Urinary losses of IgG and Factor B complement, decreased production of IgG, and nutritional deficiencies all contribute to the increased susceptibility to infection by encapsulated organisms.
Prevention	Immunization against pneumococcal infection may offer partial protection, although seroconversion is impaired in nephrotics. Penicillin prophylaxis should be considered, at least in children.

Further reading

Cameron JS. Clinical consequences of the nephrotic syndrome. In: Cameron S, Davison AM, Grünfeld J-P, Kerr DNS, Ritz E (eds) *Oxford Textbook of Clinical Nephrology*. Oxford: Oxford University Press, 1992; 276–97.
Zuchelli P. Renal vein thrombosis. *Nephrology, Dialysis and Transplantation*, 1992; **7** (Suppl. 1): 105–8.

Related topics of interest

Glomerulonephritis: general approach (p. 81)
Imaging of the urinary tract (p. 110)
Membranous nephropathy (p. 117)
Renal involvement in amyloidosis (p. 167)
Renal involvement in connective tissue diseases (p. 171)

DEVELOPMENTAL ABNORMALITIES OF THE KIDNEY

These are common, affecting up to 10% of the population and accounting for about 33% of all developmental abnormalities. Clinical manifestations vary from incidental findings to abnormalities incompatible with life. More severe abnormalities are often associated with severe abnormalities of other systems.

Aetiology
- Many anomalies can be explained if the normal development of the kidney *in utero* is understood. The metanephric kidney develops as a result of mutual induction between the mesenchyme of the metanephrogenic cap and the ascending ureteric bud. This mutual induction is associated with expression of the *WT1* gene. Tubular elements arise from epithelial cells in both of these structures. The developing kidneys and ureters subsequently migrate up the posterior abdominal wall.
- Most developmental abnormalities arise due to failure of differentiation, division or migration of these structures.
- Some abnormalities are genetically determined. Others result from *in utero* drug administration, infection or mechanical factors.

Problems
- Many abnormalities are not of clinical significance, unless complicated by infection or obstruction.
- Certain abnormalities carry a high risk of complications, ultimately leading to impaired renal function.
- Abnormalities occurring as part of syndromes affecting other organs may not be the dominant clinical problem.

Diagnosis
- The presence of a single umbilical artery, anomalies of the external genitalia or deformities of the limbs should prompt the search for anomalies of the kidney or renal tract.
- Oligohydramnios (if the fetal urine is diminished) often produces characteristic deformities of the

face, with low-set ears, a receding chin and a 'parrot-beak' nose, known as Potter's facies.
- Intravenous urography is the most frequently used investigation to define anomalies further. Renal biopsy is necessary in certain conditions.

Anomalies of renal mass
- Bilateral agenesis is incompatible with life and often associated with pulmonary hypoplasia and syringomyelia. Failure of the ureteric bud to develop, or failure of the mutual induction between ureteric bud and metanephrogenic cap, is the underlying problem.
- Unilateral agenesis of kidney, ureter and ipsilateral trigone is associated with compensatory hypertrophy of the contralateral kidney. This is rarely detected unless a super-added problem occurs.
- Renal hypoplasia is relatively uncommon. A small, poorly developed kidney with fewer calices and papillae than usual is found, often in association with ectopic or duplex ureters. Urinary salt-wasting and acidosis occur.
- Oligomeganephronia is a form of hypoplasia in which a very small kidney has a reduced number of nephrons but with large glomeruli and hypertrophy of the proximal tubules. Chronic renal failure occurs.
- Dysplasia occurs if there has been abnormal differentiation and organization of the developing kidney. The kidney is small and misshapen. On biopsy, tubules are found to be dilated and deformed with a lining of undifferentiated cells. Bizarre tissues (cartilage, smooth muscle) may be found within the kidney. This condition may be focal and coexisting with normal renal tissue – the relative proportions determine whether renal failure occurs. This condition is commonly associated with anomalies of the lower urinary tract, such as ureterocele or urethral valves. In a proportion of patients with vesico-ureteric reflux, associated renal 'scarring' may in fact be renal dysplasia.

Anomalies of migration/ rotation

- Abnormalities of the ascent up the posterior abdominal wall of the ureteric bud or of its division are common.
- Ectopic kidneys are usually found at the pelvic brim and are malrotated (the hilum faces forward in the earlier phase of development). The associated short ureter may be prone to kinking and lead to obstruction or infection. In the uncommon condition of crossed ectopia, one kidney crosses the midline and its upper pole fuses with the lower pole of its contralateral partner.
- Horseshoe kidney occurs when the lower poles of both kidneys fuse and cannot ascend past the inferior mesenteric artery.

Duplex systems and ectopic ureter

- Bifid pelvis and ureter are systems where a single ureter enters the bladder after reunion below the kidney. Abnormal peristalsis may predispose to dilatation, obstruction and infection.
- Double ureters develop if two ureteric buds have existed. The ectopic ureter enters the bladder below and medial to the normal ureter and drains the upper moiety of the kidney. This moiety may be dysplastic or hypoplasic. Either ureteric orifice may be abnormal with potential for vesico-ureteric reflux.

Obstructive lesions

- These can lead to incomplete or total obstruction of the urinary tract and include pelvi-ureteric junction obstruction, congenital megaureter, ureterocele and urethral valves. About 20% of childhood renal failure is due to obstructive lesions.

Further reading

Rascher W, Meyer-Schwickerath M, Obling H. Congenital anomalies of the urinary tract. In: Cameron JS, Davison AM, Grünfeld J-P, Kerr D, Ritz E (eds) *Oxford Textbook of Clinical Nephrology*. Oxford: Oxford University Press, 1992; 2023–43.

Related topics of interest

DIABETIC NEPHROPATHY

Diabetic nephropathy is one of the major causes of renal failure in patients starting dialysis treatment. Patients who have survived diabetes for long enough to develop nephropathy have usually developed other microvascular and macrovascular complications, and therefore pose major management problems. Prevention of diabetic nephropathy and its progression is of major importance in the management of diabetic patients.

Risk factors

1. Family history of essential hypertension. Raised red cell sodium–lithium countertransport may be a marker for increased risk.

2. Poor glycaemic control. Some evidence exists for a 'threshold' effect at a HbA1 of around 8%, although this is disputed.

3. Smoking. This also increases the risk of retinopathy.

4. Hyperlipidaemia. This is associated with more rapid progression once nephropathy is established.

Epidemiology

Cumulative risk is probably similar in type 1 (IDDM) and type 2 (NIDDM) diabetes. Type 2 diabetics may present with established nephropathy, having had undiagnosed diabetes for years before diagnosis. Only 30–40% of diabetics ever develop nephropathy. After 25 years of diabetes, the probability of the appearance of clinical nephropathy declines. The incidence is particularly high in Nordic countries; the reason for this is unclear.

Pathology

The renal lesion is characterized by increased deposition or decreased degradation of mesangial extracellular matrix, culminating in obliteration of the glomerulus and sclerosis. The following sequence is characteristic:

- Increased glomerular basement membrane thickness.
- Glomerular and tubular hypertrophy.

- Increased deposition of mesangial matrix.
- Hyalinization of arterioles.
- Progressive mesangial sclerosis culminating in nodular glomerulosclerosis ('Kimmelsteil–Wilson' nephropathy).

Clinical evolution

The following sequence is observed:

- Increased glomerular filtration rate.
- Increased excretion of albumin and other proteins.
- Systemic hypertension.
- Gradual decline in glomerular filtration rate, often at around 10 ml/min/yr, until endstage renal failure occurs.
- Accelerated coronary and peripheral vascular disease.

Structure and function

The relationship between structural changes on renal biopsy and functional changes is poor. Basement membrane thickening on renal biopsy does not correlate with the presence of nephropathy; the later changes of mesangial expansion and sclerosis are always seen in patients with nephropathy, but may occur in patients with minimal clinical evidence of disease.

Diagnosis

Early diagnosis requires detection of increased albumin excretion below the level detected by routine urinalysis – so-called 'microalbuminuria'. Options include:

- Measurement of albumin : creatinine ratio.
- Measurement of albumin excretion rate on a timed overnight or 24 h urine collection.
- Measurement of albumin concentration (either in the laboratory or with stix tests) in an early morning urine sample.

As nephropathy progresses, proteinuria becomes detectable using routine urinalysis.

Associated problems

1. Cardiovascular risk factors. These cluster in patients with nephropathy (even the earliest stages), including:

- Increased fibrinogen.
- Increased LDL and decreased HDL cholesterol.
- Increased lipoprotein (a).
- Hypertriglyceridaemia.

2. Hyporeninaemic hypoaldosteronism. This is common in diabetic nephropathy and may cause hyperkalaemia.

3. Retinopathy. This is nearly, but not always, found in patients with diabetic nephropathy. Certainly, the absence of retinopathy should raise the question of the coexistence of another renal disease.

4. Autonomic and peripheral neuropathy. These are frequently present. The distinction between diabetic and uraemic neuropathy can sometimes only be resolved by a trial of dialysis or of renal transplantation.

5. Macrovascular disease. This is common, and often clinically silent. There is good evidence that coronary artery bypass grafting of patients with endstage diabetic nephropathy awaiting renal transplantation improves their prognosis, even if no symptoms are present.

Primary prevention

The Diabetes Control and Complications Trial showed that both the development of 'microalbuminuria' and the progression to overt proteinuria are reduced by tight diabetic control in type 1 diabetes. This reduction in risk is bought at the expense of a significantly higher risk of severe hypoglycaemia. Tight control required a level of intensive education and support not likely to be reproduced in many diabetic clinics. The question of whether tight glycaemic control reduces the risk of nephropathy in type 2 diabetes will be answered by the UK Prospective Diabetes Study.

Management

The earlier stages of nephropathy appear to be more reversible than the later stages, at least as assessed by urine albumin excretion. Several interventions reduce albumin excretion in diabetic nephropathy, although it is not known whether this is accompanied by regression of the histological changes.

1. Tight diabetic control. This is of benefit, at least in 'preclinical' nephropathy.

2. Control of hypertension. This is the most important aspect of management of diabetic nephropathy. Reduction of blood pressure reduces proteinuria and has been shown in retrospective studies to be associated with a slower rate of decline of renal function. Angiotensin–converting enzyme (ACE) inhibitors are the drugs of choice in most patients, for the following reasons:

- Thiazides and β-blockers are undesirable because of their metabolic side-effects.
- For any given level of blood pressure lowering, ACE inhibitors reduce albumin excretion more than antihypertensive agents of other classes. In addition, ACE inhibitors, even in normotensive patients, retard the progression from microalbuminuria to clinical nephropathy and reduce the rate of loss of creatinine clearance and incidence of endstage renal failure in patients with clinical nephropathy.

Patients receiving ACE inhibitors are at risk of hyperkalaemia, and of acute decline in renal function, especially in the presence of renal artery stenosis (a particular risk in type 2 diabetics with macrovascular disease).

Calcium-channel blockers also have theoretical advantages in nephropathy. Dihydropyridines may increase proteinuria, but have not been compared to ACE inhibitors in adequate long-term studies of type 1 diabetes. In type 2 diabetes progression is equally slowed by dihydropyridines and by ACE inhibitors. Other types of calcium-channel blocker, such as diltiazem and verapamil, share many of the advantages of ACE inhibitors.

3. Dietary restriction of protein. This slows progression of nephropathy, but is an unwelcome addition to pre-existing dietary restrictions and may cause malnutrition if used indiscriminately. Protein restriction may work by reducing renin and angiotensin levels, and might therefore be redundant in patients already receiving treatment with ACE inhibitors.

4. Other cardiovascular risk factors. These should be controlled carefully, although evidence that lipid-lowering treatment slows progression is not available. Aspirin should be given to reduce the risk of myocardial infarction in patients with macrovascular disease.

Further reading

Clark CM, Lee DA. Prevention and treatment of the complications of diabetes mellitus. *New England Journal of Medicine*, 1995; **332**: 1210–17.
Kasiske BL, *et al.* Effect of antihypertensive therapy on the kidney in patients with diabetes: a meta–regression analysis. *Annals of Internal Medicine*, 1993; **118**: 129–38.
Lewis EJ, *et al.* The effect of angiotensin–converting–enzyme inhibition on diabetic nephropathy. *New England Journal of Medicine*, 1993; **329**: 1456–62.

Related topics of interest

DISORDERS OF DIVALENT ION METABOLISM

Hypercalcaemia

Symptoms
- Non-specific malaise, depression.
- Abdominal pain, constipation. ~muscle
- Confusion, eventually stupor. weakness,
- Polyuria, thirst, polydipsia. ↑ sleepiness.

Signs
None (but look for evidence of the underlying disease).

Causes
- Primary hyperparathyroidism is the most common cause, particularly of hypercalcaemia detected on routine screening.
- Multiple myeloma.
- Other malignancy – either caused by circulating parathyroid-related peptide (PTHrP) or by bone secondaries.
- Thyrotoxicosis.
- Sarcoidosis.
- Immobilization.
- Iatrogenic – causes include thiazide diuretics, vitamin D derivatives +/– calcium supplements.
- Milk-alkali syndrome: chronic over-use of calcium-containing antacids.
- Rebound following rhabdomyolysis.
- Familial hypocalciuria/hypercalcaemia.

Investigation
Many causes will be identified from the history and examination alone. Specific investigations include serum PTH, urine and serum electrophoresis, serum thyroxine, serum PTHrP, serum ACE and/or tissue biopsies for sarcoidosis.

Management
Treat the underlying cause. Acute hypercalcaemia should be treated with saline replacement and loop diuretics (which promote calcium and sodium excretion). Intravenous diphosphonates (e.g. sodium pamidronate) can be given to decrease bone

Acute – 20ml 10% Ca-gluconate IV over 10mins followed by
infusion of 6gm Ca-gluconate in 500ml N/S over 4-6hrs.

resorption. Mithramycin and calcitonin are less effective and more toxic. Corticosteroids are effective in sarcoidosis.

Hypocalcaemia

Symptoms

Neuromuscular irritability: faintness, paraesthesiae, muscle cramps, tetany.

Signs

- Chvostek's sign – tapping over facial nerve causes twitching of facial muscles.
- Trousseau's sign – inflation of cuff above diastolic pressure for 3 min causes spasm of fingers and wrist.

Causes

- Renal failure – though symptoms are rare because concurrent acidosis increases the fraction of total calcium which is ionized.
- Acute pancreatitis.
- Acute rhabdomyolysis.
- Hypoparathyroidism – associated with calcification of basal ganglia.
- Pseudohypoparathyroidism – a syndrome of resistance to parathyroid hormone associated with short metacarpals and extraosseous calcification. (NB. the skeletal changes can occur without the biochemical abnormalities, so-called pseudo–pseudohypoparathyroidism.)
- Iatrogenic – following parathyroidectomy.

Investigation

- Urea and electrolytes.
- Serum amylase.
- Serum PTH (appropriately high in most causes of hypocalcaemia, inappropriately low in hypoparathyroidism and after parathyroidectomy).

Management

Intravenous calcium replacement may be necessary in severe hypocalcaemia and should preferably be given via a central line. In many patients oral treatment with calcium supplements and active vitamin D derivatives is sufficient.

Hypermagnesaemia

Symptoms and signs	Muscle weakness, respiratory paralysis and CNS depression may occur if severe (e.g. $[Mg^{2+}] > 2$ mmol/l).
Causes	Impaired excretion in acute or chronic renal failure, associated with increased intake, e.g. magnesium-containing antacids.
Treatment	Treatment is similar to that of hyperkalaemia: intravenous calcium gluconate to combat the neuromuscular and cardiac depression, and dextrose and insulin to increase uptake into cells. Haemodialysis against a low-magnesium dialysate may be required.

Hypomagnesaemia

Symptoms and signs	As with hypocalcaemia, increased neuromuscular irritability may occur. Hypomagnesaemia also causes renal potassium and calcium wasting.
Causes	Increased gastrointestinal losses occur with diarrhoea (including purgative abuse) and malabsorption; increased renal losses occur with diuretic use and tubular damage.
Treatment	Precipitating agents should be withdrawn. Symptomatic hypomagnesaemia should be treated with Mg at no greater than 1 mmol/h: 50–60 mmol may be necessary over 48 h.

Hyperphosphataemia

Symptoms and signs	A high serum phosphate normally causes no symptoms but may be associated with itching. There are no physical signs.
Causes	• Renal failure: decreased renal excretion of phosphate together with hyperparathyroidism (which increases release from bone) both

contribute (whereas if renal function is normal, PTH increases phosphate excretion).

- Increased release from cells: tumour lysis syndrome, acute rhabdomyolysis.
- Exogenous: for example phosphate enema.

Treatment

Phosphate removal by dialysis is relatively inefficient, and control of hyperphosphataemia is therefore a major problem in the management of chronic renal failure. Absorption of phosphate from food can be decreased by administration of $CaCO_3$, $Mg(OH)_2$ or $Al(OH)_3$ at the start of meals: these compounds form insoluble complexes with phosphate. Early prophylaxis and treatment of hyperparathyroidism may help.

Hypophosphataemia

Symptoms and signs

Mild degrees (e.g. serum PO_4 <0.4 mmol/l) are asymptomatic. Severe hypophosphataemia causes muscle weakness, including decreased cardiac contractility and diaphragmatic weakness, as well as confusion, hallucinations and convulsions. Severe muscle damage may cause rhabdomyolysis.

Causes

- Primary hyperparathyroidism, and persistent parathyroid activity following renal transplantation.
- Refeeding after starvation (e.g. TPN after prolonged ileus).
- Rise in pH, for example treatment of acidosis (e.g. ketoacidosis), respiratory alkalosis.
- Alcoholism.

Treatment

- Acute severe hypophosphataemia: 9 mmol phosphate intravenously over 12 h, with precautions to avoid iatrogenic hypocalcaemia.
- Chronic hypophosphataemia: correct underlying cause. Oral phosphate supplements can be given if warranted but the patient should be treated rather than the blood test.

Further reading

Bilezikian JP. Management of acute hypercalcaemia. *New England Journal of Medicine*, 1992; **326**: 1196–203.

Nussbaum SR. Pathophysiology and management of severe hypercalcaemia. *Endocrinology and Metabolism Clinics of North America*, 1993; **22**: 343–62.

Reber PM. Hypocalcaemic emergencies. *Medical Clinics of North America*, 1995; **79**: 93–106.

Related topics of interest

DISORDERS OF EXTRACELLULAR VOLUME

Water accounts for 50–60% of the weight of a normal subject – less if the subject is obese (as fat contains little water). Of this, approximately two-thirds is intracellular and the remainder extracellular. Blood volume accounts for a small proportion of extracellular fluid, the rest being interstitial. The body controls extracellular volume by controlling the excretion of its dominant cation – sodium. Distribution of fluid between the interstitial and vascular space is determined by the balance between hydrostatic and oncotic pressures in the vascular and interstitial spaces. Disorders of the amount and distribution of extracellular fluid may therefore be caused by disorders of sodium handling, cardiac function, capillary permeability, lymphatic function or serum albumin concentration.

Increased extracellular volume

Signs

The presence of clinically detectable oedema indicates retention of at least 2 l of sodium and water. This is true whatever the cause of oedema formation. Oedema of recent onset is 'pitting', whereas long-standing oedema (usually due to lymphoedema) is 'non-pitting'.

Nephrotic syndrome

Heavy proteinuria causes both hypoalbuminaemia and renal sodium retention. Together these cause oedema formation, which may be massive. Oedema is widely distributed and may vary with posture. Facial and upper limb oedema are characteristic, and are particularly obvious after recumbency. Ascites and pleural effusions are often seen.

Because of the sodium retention, circulating volume may remain normal despite the tendency for fluid to leave the vascular space as a result of decreased oncotic pressure. However, diuretic treatment results in decreased circulating volume and may precipitate pre-renal renal impairment.

Cardiac failure

Cardiac failure causes renal sodium retention and increased venous pressure. Together these cause oedema. Increased right atrial pressure results in peripheral oedema and in ascites and pleural effusions; increased left atrial pressure causes pulmonary oedema.

Chronic renal failure

Chronic renal failure is often associated with a degree of sodium retention which may cause hypertension, oedema or both. In endstage renal failure, inadequate removal of fluid by dialysis together with excessive salt and water intake leads to peripheral oedema.

Local causes

Oedema may accumulate as a result of a local increase in hydrostatic pressure, as in lower-limb oedema complicating venous insufficiency or lymphatic obstruction. Local increases in capillary permeability to proteins, resulting in loss of the normal transcapillary oncotic pressure gradient, may also cause oedema formation – as in bee stings and in cellulitis.

Third spaces

Large amounts of fluid can accumulate outside the normal circulating volume, usually as a result of local disease states but sometimes as a result of a generalized increase in permeability (e.g. ovarian hyperstimulation syndrome):

- ascites;
- pleural effusions;
- pericardial effusions.

Mobilization of fluid from these spaces may be very difficult, even when the initiating cause has been corrected.

Hypovolaemia

Signs

Decreased interstitial fluid causes loss of skin turgor; decreased circulating volume causes low jugular venous pressure and postural hypotension. Dryness of the mouth is a sign of mouth breathing and is of no use in the assessment of fluid balance. Signs of hypovolaemia in a patient with oedema should prompt a search for local causes of oedema.

Sodium wasting	Inappropriate renal excretion of sodium despite hypovolaemia is most often caused by inappropriate diuretic therapy. It may also occur after relief of obstruction, and less commonly in reflux nephropathy.
Addison's disease	Mineralocorticoid deficiency causes failure of renal sodium retention in exchange for potassium.

Further reading

Schrier RW. Body fluid volume regulation in health and disease: a unifying hypothesis. *Annals of Internal Medicine*, 1990; **113**: 155-9.

Tomson CRV. Focus on physiology and pathophysiology of fluids and electrolytes: basic principles. *Current Anaesthesia and Critical Care*, 1996; **7** (4):176–181.

Related topics of interest

Acute renal failure: general approach (p. 11)
Dysnatraemias (p. 70)
Glomerulonephritis: general approach (p. 81)

DRUG-INDUCED RENAL DISEASE

Many drugs can lead directly or indirectly to renal dysfunction. It is critical to identify possible risk factors for drug-induced renal disease in individual patients before any act of prescription. The usual clinical problem is acute renal failure (ARF) but chronic renal syndromes may also be caused by drugs.

Problems

- A variety of heterogeneous clinical syndromes occur.
- The incidence of drug-induced renal disease continues to increase. Drugs are implicated as the principal cause of ARF in up to 20% of cases. They contribute with other renal insults in many other cases.
- ECF volume depletion and electrolyte abnormalities, especially hypokalaemia and hypomagnesaemia, are important risk factors for the development of drug-induced ARF.
- Ischaemic acute tubular necrosis (ATN) due to alterations in intra-renal haemodynamics occurs with non-steroidal anti-inflammatory drugs (NSAIDs), angiotensin-converting enzyme inhibitors (ACEIs) and cyclosporin.
- Toxic ATN occurs with the use of aminoglycosides, amphotericin, cisplatin and foscarnet. Overdoses of paracetamol cause ARF by a similar mechanism.
- Acute allergic interstitial nephritis (AIN) has been reported with a vast number of drugs, but especially NSAIDs, β-lactam antibiotics, captopril, rifampicin, allopurinol, ciprofloxacin, and sulphonamides.
- ARF with intratubular crystallization and obstruction can occur with intravenous acyclovir and trimethoprim–sulphamethoxazole (co-trimoxazole).
- CRF with chronic interstitial nephritis (CIN) occurs with NSAIDs, cyclosporin, lithium, nitrosoureas and cisplatin.
- Analgesic nephropathy, a specific syndrome of CIN, occurs with long-term use of compound analgesic preparations.

- Immune complex-mediated glomerulopathies are classically associated with gold and penicillamine therapy but have been reported with many other drugs.

NSAIDs

- Most patients taking NSAIDs suffer no clinical renal problems. Experimental studies do show alterations in renal excretion of prostaglandins and in the renal handling of sodium and potassium even in normal subjects.
- NSAIDs may antagonize the action of anti-hypertensive drugs, particularly diuretics.
- Idiosyncratic acute allergic interstitial nephritis, presenting as ARF, has been reported frequently but is not a common event.
- NSAIDs are very important causes of ARF in a particular subset of patients, and are now probably the group of drugs most frequently implicated in hospital-acquired ARF.
- Afferent arteriolar blood flow is normally sensitive to, but not dependent upon, the action of prostaglandins. In patients with long-standing cardiac failure, hepatic failure or renal failure this autoregulation is dependent upon the action of prostaglandins.
- If these patients become ECF volume depleted or suffer some other derangement of the circulation, then continued or new administration of NSAIDs inhibits the production of prostaglandins and allows vasoconstrictive factors to act unopposed. The presenting feature of this is oligo-anuric ARF. Characteristically this occurs in elderly patients with a number of risk factors for the development of ARF.
- Withdrawal of the drug and the usual supportive measures for ARF are indicated. Renal replacement therapy may be necessary.
- NSAIDs are also common causes of hyperkalaemic distal RTA.
- NSAIDs may cause nephrotic syndrome: renal biopsy shows minimal glomerular abnormality, but a patchy interstitial infiltrate.

ACEIs

- ARF is relatively uncommon when all patients treated by ACEIs are considered. It is more likely in patients with renal artery stenosis, but also occurs in ECF volume-depleted patients and in those with poor left ventricular function, cirrhosis, pre-existing renal impairment or diffuse vascular disease.
- Renin and angiotensin maintain the efferent arteriolar tone. If afferent arteriolar pressures drop (across a stenosis, for example) then the intraglomerular pressure and, hence the glomerular filtration rate, can only be maintained by efferent arteriolar constriction. Interference with this mechanism by ACEIs causes an acute drop in GFR.
- Non-oliguric or oliguric ARF occurs. Frequently this is quickly reversible on discontinuing the drug, but protracted dialysis-requiring ARF may follow, especially in vulnerable elderly patients.
- ACEIs are also common causes of hyperkalaemic distal RTA.

Aminoglycosides

- Even in optimal circumstances, ARF occurs in 5–7% of patients taking these drugs. The proportion increases in the presence of risk factors such as increasing age, ECF volume depletion, hypokalaemia, hypomagnesaemia, co-administration of other nephrotoxins and pre-existing renal impairment.
- These are highly cationic drugs which bind to negatively charged phosphatidylinositol on the cell membrane of the proximal tubule. Bound tissue levels are 10–20 times higher than circulating plasma levels. Tissue uptake is saturable at high plasma concentrations and is lowest for once daily treatment.
- Non-oliguric ARF with an asymptomatic rise in plasma creatinine is the usual initial presentation. Marked urinary losses of potassium and magnesium may occur. Renal biopsy shows a toxic ATN.
- Withdrawal of the drug (and any other nephrotoxins), correction of ECF volume and

electrolyte problems and general supportive measures usually lead to a full recovery of renal function. It is unusual for renal replacement therapy to be necessary.

- Aminoglycosides should be prescribed only with continuing pharmacokinetic assessment of trough and peak plasma levels, particularly in high-risk patients. Once-daily dosages are preferable.

- High plasma levels of aminoglycosides occur during ARF. The inner ear is another target organ which may be damaged at this time. In contrast to renal dysfunction, such damage may be irreversible.

Amphotericin

- Over 75% of patients treated with this drug exhibit an asymptomatic rise in plasma creatinine. ECF volume depletion is the most important risk factor. Saline-loading prior to administration is desirable. Hypokalaemia and hypomagnesaemia are also risk factors.

- The earliest signs of toxicity are loss of urinary concentrating ability and increased urinary excretion of potassium and magnesium.

- This drug has a complex mechanism of toxicity. It complexes with sterols in cell membranes, disrupting and increasing their permeability. It also affects afferent and efferent arteriolar blood flow, leading to ischaemia. There is some evidence to suggest that liposomal preparations of amphotericin are less toxic.

- It is important to recognize that amphotericin may be life-saving in a patient with fungal sepsis, and that fungal sepsis itself is a potent cause of ARF.

Cyclosporin

- Cyclosporin can cause acute reversible nephrotoxicity due to vasoconstriction of afferent and efferent arterioles, with decreased renal blood flow and glomerular filtration rate. This is frequently seen with higher doses. Prior administration of calcium-entry blockers attenuates this effect.

- Chronic administration of cyclosporin, especially in heart and liver transplant recipients, causes an obliterative arteriolopathy with a characteristic striped interstitial fibrosis. This causes progressive CRF and is largely irreversible.
- It also acts as a direct tubular toxin, causing hyperkalaemia, impaired urinary concentrating ability and hypophosphataemia.

Paracetamol

- If taken in excess, as in self-poisoning, paracetamol may lead to ARF. Hepatic damage is common in this context, but occasionally renal damage is the more prominent clinical manifestation.
- Most paracetamol is freely filtered (10–15% is protein-bound); 60–70% is reabsorbed in the proximal tubule. It is preferentially metabolized to glucuronyl and sulphate conjugates and subsequently excreted. When this system becomes saturated, the unconjugated drug is metabolized by the cytochrome P450 mixed oxidase system. When, in turn, this system becomes saturated, there is a build up of reactive metabolites which bind to and induce cellular injury.
- Focal tubular necrosis occurs with focal vascular injury to the kidney. Recovery is usual, provided that the patient recovers from the associated hepatic injury.

Further reading

Fillastre JP, Godin M. Drug-induced nephropathies. In: Cameron JS, Davison AM, Grünfeld J-P, Kerr D, Ritz E (eds) *Oxford Textbook of Clinical Nephrology*. Oxford: Oxford University Press, 1992; 159–75.

Paller MS. Drug-induced nephropathies. *Medical Clinics of North America*, 1990, **74**: 909–17.

Related topics of interest

DYSKALAEMIAS

Disorders of plasma potassium concentration are common occurrences, with potentially serious consequences, including dysrythmias and sudden cardiac death.

Normal potassium homeostasis

- Total body potassium content is about 50 mmol/kg Most is intracellular (140–150 mmol/l), primarily in muscle. Two per cent of total body potassium is in the extracellular fluid (3.5–5.0 mmol/l).
- Normal dietary intake is about 0.75 to 1.5 mmol/kg/day. Children have higher requirements, as do adults participating in vigorous exercise. Minimum intake of 20–30 mmol/day is needed to avoid significant depletion. Up to 500 mmol/day can be excreted in the urine in the face of a high dietary intake.
- The intracellular:extracellular potassium ratio is dependent on the membrane Na^+/K^+-ATPase activity. Activity of this enzyme is affected by H^+ balance, plasma tonicity, and plasma insulin, adrenaline and aldosterone concentrations.
- Acute potassium homeostasis is largely regulated by shifts between the intracellular and extracellular compartments. Although a small amount of potassium is excreted in faeces, the kidney is the principal organ responsible for chronic potassium homeostasis.

Renal excretion of potassium

- Ninety per cent of filtered potassium is reabsorbed in the proximal tubule. Usually no more than 10% reaches the distal tubule. Potassium secretion occurs from the principal cells in the mid- and late-distal tubule and in the cortical collecting duct. Potassium absorption occurs principally in the outer medullary collecting duct.
- During dietary potassium restriction, potassium secretion is suppressed and there is net potassium absorption. The converse applies in the case of excessive potassium intake or hyperkalaemia.
- Potassium is pumped into tubular cells from the peritubular capillaries by an active mechanism loosely coupled with apical sodium absorption.

Secretion into the tubular lumen is via conductive potassium channels and by a potassium–chloride co-transporter.

- Potassium secretion is enhanced by aldosterone, hyperkalaemia and acute metabolic acidosis. Increased urine flow rates, increased sodium delivery and decreased chloride delivery to the distal tubule all stimulate net potassium secretion.
- Potassium absorption is linked to H^+-secretion by a luminal H^+/K^+-ATPase. The activity of this pump is dependent on dietary potassium intake, luminal sodium concentration and arterial pCO_2. Acute respiratory acidosis increases the activity of the pump, leading to a decrease in net urinary potassium excretion, with acute respiratory alkalosis acting in the opposite direction.

Extrarenal homeostasis

- Metabolic acidosis increases plasma potassium, with an increment of about 0.6 mmol/l (range 0.2–1.7 mmol/l) for each decrease of 0.1 pH units. Respiratory acidosis has a considerably less marked effect with an increment of 0.1 mmol/l per 0.1 pH unit. Similarly, metabolic alkalosis decreases plasma potassium by about 0.3 mmol/l for each increment of 0.1 pH units, and respiratory alkalosis by about 0.25 mmol/l per 0.1 pH unit increment.
- Insulin is the most important regulator of transcellular potassium distribution, acting indirectly via the enzyme Na^+/K^+-ATPase. β-adrenergic agonists also stimulate movement of potassium into cells. These act through β_2-receptors in most tissues, except the heart where β_1-receptors mediate potassium uptake. α-adrenergic agonists cause hyperkalaemia by enhancing potassium release from the liver and decreasing uptake by skeletal muscle.
- With normal renal function, colonic excretion of potassium accounts for no more than 10% of total excretion. This proportion increases with CRF. The colon has a sensitivity to aldosterone similar to the collecting duct.

Hyperkalaemia

- Plasma [K$^+$] >5.0 mmol/l may be artefactual or real. Real hyperkalaemia reflects an altered distribution between intracellular and extracellular compartments occurring in the setting of normal or abnormal renal function.
- Usually asymptomatic. Muscle weakness or non-specific myalgia may occur. Occasionally presents as symptomatic bradycardia or sudden cardiac death.
- A sequence of ECG changes occur. Initial changes include 'tenting' of T waves. More severe elevation of [K$^+$] leads to broadening of the QRS complex and bradycardia.
- Artefactual hyperkalaemia may reflect haemolysis, severe thrombocytosis or marked leucocytosis.

Redistribution without impaired renal potassium excretion

- Rapid intravenous infusion (especially if >40 mmol/h) of large amounts of potassium can overwhelm normal homeostatic mechanisms, as can the release of massive amounts of intracellular potassium with tissue necrosis, rhabdomyolysis, tumour necrosis, retroperitoneal haemorrhage and intravascular haemolysis. Depolarizing muscle relaxants, such as succinylcholine, may have this effect especially in patients with burns, spinal cord injuries and lower motor neurone diseases. Drugs such as spironolactone, propranolol and digoxin may decrease intracellular uptake of potassium.
- Episodic acute release of cellular potassium with attacks of paralysis lasting from minutes to hours occurs in hyperkalaemic, periodic paralysis. This rare, autosomal dominant condition is due to a defect in sodium channel deactivation. β$_2$ agonists can successfully treat the acute attack. Episodes may be prevented by acetazolamide.

Redistribution with impaired renal potassium excretion

- Occurs with impaired renal function in ARF and CRF. In CRF, there is increased fractional excretion of potassium per surviving nephron, increased colonic excretion and increased intracellular distribution. In ARF there is less time for these mechanisms to develop - hyperkalaemia may be of more rapid onset and severe degree. Associated acidosis impairs intracellular redistribution.

- Hyporeninaemic hypoaldosteronism is part of the spectrum of normal ageing and is especially frequent in those with interstitial nephritis, diabetic nephropathy and chronic ECF volume expansion.
- Drugs such as NSAIDs, ACEIs, amiloride and heparin may cause hyperkalaemia, largely by causing a distal hyperkalaemic RTA.

Treatment of hyperkalaemia

- This is a life-threatening medical emergency which needs prompt and immediate therapy. Patients should be attached to a cardiac monitor with easy availability of resuscitation equipment.
- Parenteral and oral potassium supplements should be discontinued, dietary intake reviewed and offending drug therapy discontinued.
- Intravenous calcium gluconate or calcium chloride (10 ml of 10% solution; 2.25 mmol Ca^{2+}) should be given immediately to stabilize the myocardial cell membrane.
- If hyperkalaemia is severe, or there are ECG changes, i.v. insulin and dextrose may be given. A common error is to use too much insulin, thereby additionally causing hypoglycaemia. In patients without insulin resistance a ratio of 5 g carbohydrate per unit of insulin is appropriate. Thus, 50 ml of 50% dextrose contains 25 g carbohydrate and should be prescribed with 5 units of insulin. Milder cases can be treated (in non-diabetics) by i.v. glucose infusion alone, as this will stimulate endogenous insulin release.
- There is good evidence that simultaneous administration of i.v. bicarbonate (e.g. 1.26% $NaHCO_3$ solution at 50–100 ml/h) with i.v. insulin/dextrose has an additional decremental effect on plasma $[K^+]$.
- Inhaled β-agonists, such as salbutamol, will further decrease plasma $[K^+]$ by about 0.1–0.3 mmol/l.
- Polystyrene sulphonate resins such as calcium resonium act as ion exchangers in the gut. Onset of action is slow, however.

- If hyperkalaemia remains severe, especially with more advanced ECG changes and renal impairment, then dialysis therapy is necessary.

Hypokalaemia

- Usually asymptomatic, but may present with weakness and cardiac dysrythmias, especially in patients treated with digoxin.
- May reflect redistribution from extracellular to intracellular compartments, dietary deficiency, or excessive renal or extrarenal losses. Normal kidneys will decrease potassium excretion to less than 20 mmol/day in the presence of hypokalaemia.

Redistribution

- Intracellular redistribution occurs during systemic alkalaemia (which also stimulates kaliuresis) and with high catecholamine secretion as can occur in myocardial infarction, severe head injury or delirium tremens. Hypokalaemic periodic paralysis is a rare, autosomal dominant disorder with episodic bouts of profound muscle weakness and severe hypokalaemia. A similar pattern may be seen in thyrotoxicosis, especially in patients of Oriental origin. Barium, toluene and theophylline poisoning cause intracellular redistribution.

Excessive renal potassium losses

- Associated with hypertension in mineralocorticoid and glucocorticoid excess and with diuretic therapy. Also with adrenal enzyme defects (11 β-hydroxylase and 17 α-hydroxylase deficiencies) and accelerated hypertension with associated hyperreninaemia.
- Associated with normotension and metabolic acidosis in DKA, ureterosigmoidostomy, RTA and use of acetazolamide.
- Associated with normotension and metabolic alkalosis in prolonged vomiting, nasogastric suction and Barrter's syndrome.
- Associated with normotension and normal acid–base status in interstitial nephritis, diuretic phase of ATN, post-obstructive diuresis,

magnesium depletion and use of drugs such as aminoglycosides and cisplatin.

- Loss of upper GI fluid from vomiting and nasogastric suction causes depletion of fluid and hydrochloric acid, but little potassium loss. However, the resulting metabolic alkalosis results in renal potassium wasting and thus in hypokalaemia.

Excessive extrarenal potassium losses

- Diarrhoea, in contrast, results in significant GI potassium losses and, frequently, in metabolic acidosis. Hypokalaemia in this situation reflects GI losses despite renal conservation of potassium.

Treatment of hypokalaemia

- Offending drugs should be discontinued and specific therapy given for any identifiable underlying defect. Chloride-responsive metabolic alkalosis should be corrected.
- Increased dietary intake should be promoted. This may need to be augmented by oral potassium supplements. In patients with significant depletion, large amounts (>100 mmol/day) may be needed to correct the deficit. Potassium should not be given more rapidly than 10 mmol/h i.v., even with significant depletion. Especial care to avoid hyperkalaemia is needed if renal function is impaired.
- Resistant hypokalaemia should prompt that magnesium deficiency be excluded or corrected as appropriate.

Further reading

Tannen RL. Hypo-hyperkalaemia. In: Cameron JS, Davison AM, Grünfeld J-P, Kerr D, Ritz E (eds) *Oxford Textbook of Clinical Nephrology*. Oxford: Oxford University Press, 1992; 895–916.

Related topics of interest

DYSNATRAEMIAS

Disturbances of plasma sodium concentration are found in a variety of disease states. Sodium is the principal solute contributing to the effective plasma osmolality (tonicity). Because of the intimate association between sodium and water balance, disorders of plasma sodium concentration must always be evaluated in the context of the prevailing state of hydration of the extracellular and intracellular fluid compartments. Dysnatraemias are best regarded as disorders of water balance rather than sodium balance.

Regulation of water balance

- Water excretion is largely under the control of plasma antidiuretic hormone (ADH) which is released by the posterior pituitary in response to a number of osmotic and non-osmotic stimuli.
- Plasma osmolality normally ranges from 280 to 295 mosm/kg. This is the main influence on ADH release. If plasma osmolality rises, ADH secretion increases. ADH then acts on the renal tubule to increase solute-free water reabsorption and restore normal plasma osmolality. The converse occurs when plasma osmolality falls.
- ECF volume depletion is a potent non-osmotic stimulus to ADH release. If an ECF volume contraction of 4% or more has occurred, ADH release will continue, whatever the plasma osmolality, until the ECF volume deficit has been corrected.
- Nausea and signals from the oropharynx contribute to ADH release. A number of drugs modify its secretion and its action on the tubule.
- Thirst controls water intake. Thirst is a complex mechanism responding to osmotic and non-osmotic stimuli, including afferent signals from baroreceptors and levels of circulating angiotensin II.
- The kidney can excrete a small volume of concentrated ($\geq$1000 mosm/kg) urine or a large volume (up to 15 l/day) of very dilute (50 mosm/kg) urine in response to different clinical circumstances.
- The ability to excrete solute-free water is the principal mechanism protecting against

hyponatraemia. Impairment of this mechanism is thus the principal underlying problem in hyponatraemic states.

- An inadequate thirst mechanism or inadequate access to water, rather than an impaired ability by the kidney to conserve water, is the usual underlying problem in hypernatraemic states.

Renal conservation of solute-free water

- In the face of disorders which threaten to create cellular dehydration and hypernatraemia, the kidney will conserve solute-free water.
- In the proximal tubule, water is reabsorbed, primarily with solute absorption, through aquaporin-1 water channels.
- Some reabsorption of solute-free water occurs in the thin descending limb of the loop of Henle in response to the surrounding medullary tonicity.
- The thick ascending limb of the loop of Henle (TALH) permits active solute reabsorption, via the $Na^+-K^+-2Cl^-$ co-transporter, but is impermeable to water. This is the 'diluting' segment of the nephron. More importantly, by active transport of solute out of the nephron, the medullary thick ascending limb of the loop of Henle (MTALH) generates the hypertonic medullary interstitium. This creates the osmotic gradient for solute-free water absorption from other sites along the nephron.
- Maintenance of the hypertonic medullary gradient thus requires an adequate delivery of sodium and chloride to the MTALH. In addition, sufficient urea delivery is required to allow the 'countercurrent multiplier' effect to continue.
- ADH acts on the collecting duct via the V_2 receptor. Activation of this leads to the insertion of the aquaporin-2 water channel across the membrane of this normally impermeable section of the nephron. Solute-free water reabsorption then occurs, driven by the medullary interstitial osmotic gradient.
- Normal renal architecture, intact MTALH function and normal ADH effect are thus necessary to allow renal conservation of water.

Renal excretion of solute-free water

- In the face of disorders which threaten to create cellular overhydration and hyponatraemia, the kidney will excrete solute-free water.
- Urine cannot be rendered completely solute-free as there is a minimum obligatory osmolar load of 700 mosm to be excreted.
- The mechanisms governing solute-free water excretion are similar, but not identical, to those governing solute-free water conservation.
- Increased solute-free water excretion requires a normal renal blood flow, normal glomerular filtration rate, intact TALH function, minimum ADH effect and normal osmolar solute excretion. Reduced medullary tonicity is also important.

Classification of dysnatraemias

- Dysnatraemias should be classified by considering the direction and magnitude of the abnormality in plasma sodium concentration, the prevailing ECF volume status, the duration of the problem and the presence of symptoms.
- In chronic dysnatraemias there has been sufficient time for cerebral adaptation to occur by loss/gain of low molecular weight organic osmoles. Rapid correction of dysnatraemia in this context may lead to acute cerebral events, as de-adaptation may take several days.

Acute hyponatraemic syndromes

- These are usually caused by administration of excessive hypotonic fluids in circumstances where the renal ability to excrete free water may be impaired. Because of rapid onset (<48 h), cerebral oedema may occur. Frequently symptomatic with confusion, seizures, respiratory arrest and coma. Unless treated promptly, these may lead to death or permanent neurological abnormalities.
- Post-operative hyponatraemia (<130 mmol/l) occurs in up to 5% of patients. Surgery and anaesthesia are non-osmotic stimuli to ADH release. Pre-operative fasting decreases urinary solute excretion. Absorption of the irrigating fluid used in transurethral prostatectomy may occur, with symptomatic acute hyponatraemia,

especially if sorbitol- or glycine-containing fluids are used.

- Oxytocin infusion to induce delivery, in conjunction with i.v. infusion of hypotonic fluid, may cause acute hyponatraemia because of its ADH-like effects. Intravenous cyclophosphamide infusion does not alter ADH levels, but may alter the permeability of the collecting duct to water. If large volumes of oral or i.v. fluids are concurrently administered to reduce the risk of haemorrhagic cystitis, and if the patient has some degree of renal impairment, then acute symptomatic hyponatraemia is a possible adverse event.

- Psychotic patients may develop acute hyponatraemia after episodes of compulsive water drinking. Frequently, an associated abnormality limiting the ability of the kidney to excrete solute-free water will be found, such as prescription of drugs enhancing ADH release.

- If hyponatraemia is of abrupt onset, there is insufficient time for cellular adaptation and the risk of cerebral oedema is high. Treatment with hypertonic saline is indicated in this situation. The risks of neurological damage outweigh the risk of rapid correction of hyponatraemia. Such patients should be treated in an intensive care unit. After inducing a diuresis with frusemide they should be infused with that volume of 3% saline that contains the same amount of sodium (mmol) as is being excreted in the urine over the same time interval, until the $[Na^+]$ has increased by 10%. Correction should not exceed 20 mmol/day.

Chronic hyponatraemia with increased ECF volume

- This occurs in chronic oedematous states such as cardiac failure, cirrhosis with ascites or nephrotic syndrome.

- In these conditions there is a decreased 'effective arterial volume'. This leads to a decrease in GFR with increased proximal fluid reabsorption, further enhanced by increased renal sympathetic nerve activity and secondary hyperaldosteronism.

There is decreased filtrate delivery to the MTALH diluting segment. The apparent decrease in effective arterial blood volume is also a potent non-osmotic stimulus to ADH release. All these derangements impair the ability to excrete solute-free water.

- Loop diuretics may contribute to the problem by further interfering with MTALH function. Paradoxically, and especially if used with ACEIs, they may have a net beneficial effect by increasing delivery of filtrate to the MTALH.
- Treatment consists of cautious use of loop diuretic agents, avoidance of excessive hypotonic fluid intake, and optimization of cardiac output. Theoretically a combination of β-blockers, ACEIs and selective V_2 antagonists is the most rational approach, but there is little clinical experience with this.

Chronic hyponatraemia with decreased ECF volume

- ECF depletion may have occurred because of renal losses of salt, as in adrenal insufficiency, Barrter's syndrome, excessive use of diuretics and with salt-wasting nephropathies. Urinary sodium concentration is usually greater than 20 mmol/l.
- ECF depletion may have occurred because of extra-renal sodium loss as in severe diarrhoea or inflammatory bowel disease or profuse sweating. Urinary sodium excretion is usually less than 10 mmol/l.
- The mechanism of hyponatraemia is the inability to excrete solute-free water due to decreased solute delivery to the diluting section of the nephron and activation of angiotensin, renal nerves and ADH, often in the face of a high water intake.
- Treatment consists of rehydration with crystalloids, such as isotonic saline, which will allow the kidney to recover its usual functions. Some restriction of water intake may be prudent.

Chronic hyponatraemia with near normal ECF volume	• The syndrome of inappropriate ADH secretion (SIADH) is the most common euvolaemic hypotonic condition. It presents with less than maximally dilute urine in the presence of hyponatraemia, with normal renal, hepatic and cardiac function and no evident disturbance of ECF volume status.
	• SIADH is associated with a range of malignancies, especially small cell carcinoma of the lung. CNS disease, including brain tumours, brain abscesses, head injury and cerebral lupus, have been reported to cause SIADH.
	• Chlorpropramide augments ADH release from the pituitary and also enhances its action on the renal tubules. Carbamazepine enhances ADH release in a dose-dependent fashion.
Hypernatraemia	• Implies coexistent hypertonicity and intracellular volume contraction. Often not associated with clinical signs of ECF depletion unless considerable. Impaired access to water due to illness or coma is the usual reason for this. Onset is slow, allowing time for cerebral adaptation – correction should not be too rapid. Thirst declines with age. Elderly men become less thirsty with water deprivation than younger men despite a greater rise in plasma sodium concentration. Cerebral tumours, infections and degenerative lesions also interfere with thirst.
	• Hypernatraemia may occur in diabetes insipidus, but this is unusual if there is free access to fluid, unless the thirst mechanism is impaired.
	• Infusion of 8.4% bicarbonate solutions may cause hypernatraemia – this solution contains 1000 mmol Na^+/l.
Diabetes insipidus (DI)	• Presents with polyuria, inappropriately dilute urine and, sometimes, hypernatraemia. It may be central or nephrogenic. The principal differential diagnosis is with primary polydipsia. After 16 h

of water deprivation a urine osmolality of 1000 mosm/kg should be achieved. Failure to do so suggests a diagnosis of DI, which can be further characterized by the administration of exogenous desmopressin.

- ADH release is defective in central DI. Fifty per cent of cases are idiopathic. Many have circulating antibodies to ADH-secreting cells. Head trauma, pituitary surgery, brain tumours and local vascular disorders may be found. Fewer than 5% of cases are familial, showing an X-linked inheritance pattern. Intranasal desmopressin, 10–20 μg twice daily, usually controls this problem.
- Nephrogenic DI may reflect the inability to develop a hypertonic medullary interstitium or insensitivity of the collecting tubule to ADH, and may be acquired or hereditary. Acquired insensitivity to ADH may be due to hypokalaemia, hypercalcaemia or lithium, demeclocycline or amphotericin administration.

Further reading

Berl T. Treating hyponatraemia: Damned if we do and damned if we don't. *Kidney International,* 1990; **37**: 1006–18.

Gabow PA. Hypo-hypernatraemia. In: Cameron JS, Davison AM, Grünfeld J-P, Kerr D, Ritz E (eds) *Oxford Textbook of Clinical Nephrology.* Oxford: Oxford University Press, 1992; 869–94.

Schrier RW. Pathogenesis of sodium and water retention in high-output and low-output cardiac failure, nephrotic syndrome, cirrhosis and pregnancy. *New England Journal of Medicine,* 1988; **319**: 1127–34.

Related topics of interest

Disorders of extracellular volume (p. 54)
Drug-induced renal disease (p. 57)

FOCAL SEGMENTAL GLOMERULOSCLEROSIS

Many different diseases can cause focal segmental glomerulosclerosis (FSGS). A renal biopsy report of FSGS therefore needs to be interpreted in the light of other clinical information. 'Idiopathic' FSGS is one of the major causes of nephrotic syndrome in adults and children, and forms part of a spectrum with minimal change glomerulonephritis. The distinction is important because primary FSGS frequently recurs in kidney transplants and because it may respond to immunosuppressive treatment. Both forms carry a poor prognosis, with a high rate of progression to endstage renal failure.

Pathology

Light microscopy shows deposition of featureless hyaline material ('sclerosis') in parts ('segmental') of some ('focal') glomeruli. Immune reactants are absent apart from in the areas of sclerosis, where IgM and C3 are deposited, probably by non-specific trapping. Electron microscopy shows foot process fusion which may be partial or complete (complete fusion is more suggestive of 'idiopathic' or primary FSGS). Juxtamedullary glomeruli are involved first in the earlier stages, and the changes may therefore be missed in a superficial biopsy.

Some of the 'secondary' forms of FSGS have particular pathological features, such as severe tubulointerstitial scarring in heroin nephropathy and 'collapsing' global glomerulosclerosis in HIV nephropathy.

Primary FSGS

FSGS is the cause of up to 15% of cases of nephrotic syndrome in children and in a greater proportion of adults. Its incidence appears to be increasing, particularly in Afro-American males, in whom it is the most common single diagnosis in renal biopsy. It has many similarities to minimal change disease, and may be considered as part of a spectrum, with pure minimal change disease at the most benign end of the spectrum and steroid-resistant FSGS at the most severe end. Both are termed 'idiopathic nephrotic syndrome'. Patients who initially have steroid-responsive minimal change disease may later become steroid resistant and have FSGS on repeat biopsy.

Presentation	• Proteinuria, often with full-blown nephrotic syndrome. • Impaired or deteriorating renal function. • Hypertension in 30–50%.
Investigation	Proteinuria is unselective. There are no other tests, apart from renal biopsy, which allow FSGS to be differentiated from minimal change disease. Renal vein thrombosis should be considered in patients with haematuria and/or rapidly declining renal function.
Natural history	Spontaneous remission is rare. Patients presenting with asymptomatic proteinuria often progress to full–blown nephrotic syndrome, which is followed in most patients by progressive renal failure. Primary FSGS frequently recurs in transplanted kidneys, and this has been shown to be associated with a circulating protein which causes proteinuria.
Treatment	*1. Supportive.* Control of oedema may require diuretics. Hypertension should be controlled carefully. High-protein diets exacerbate proteinuria and should be avoided. As in other causes of nephrotic syndrome, consideration should be given to prophylactic anticoagulants and antibiotics. ACE inhibitors, in addition to controlling hypertension, reduce proteinuria (particularly if combined with dietary sodium restriction) and may help to control oedema. Whether ACE inhibitor-induced reduction of proteinuria improves long-term outcome remains uncertain. *2. Steroids.* Patients with FSGS do not usually respond to the steroid regimens used for minimal change disease. However, at least some patients experience a remission if treated with prolonged high-dose steroids (e.g. 60 mg/day for ≥6 months), and remission of proteinuria is associated with a greatly reduced risk of progressive renal disease. However, controlled trials have not been performed.

3. Cytotoxic agents. Uncontrolled trials have suggested that prolonged courses of cyclophosphamide or azathioprine with steroids may induce lasting remission in at least some patients. There is no way of identifying in advance 'responders' to steroid or cytotoxic treatment. As in minimal change disease, cytotoxic treatment may reduce the risk of subsequent relapse if remission is achieved.

4. Cyclosporin. As in minimal change disease, cyclosporin is not thought to induce a lasting remission but to maintain remission only for as long as the drug is used. Patients with FSGS seem particularly susceptible to cyclosporin nephrotoxicity, with worsening of glomerular lesions on repeat renal biopsy.

Secondary FSGS

Glomerulosclerosis is the final result of many different causes of glomerular injury, and is freqently focal and segmental. These causes must be differentiated from primary FSGS, because both the natural history and response to treatment are entirely different.

Causes

- Late stage of focal glomerulonephritis.
- Remnant nephropathy. Any disease resulting in loss of significant numbers of nephrons can cause progressive sclerosis in the remaining glomeruli, probably as a consequence of maladaptive hyperfiltration and hypertrophy of the remaining nephrons. FSGS can therefore be seen in patients with renal dysplasia, reflux nephropathy or surgical loss of renal mass.
- Sickle-cell disease can cause a number of glomerular lesions, including membranous nephropathy; FSGS in these patients may represent a form of remnant nephropathy following sickling damage.
- Obesity.
- Cyanotic heart disease.

- Heroin abuse.
- HIV nephropathy.
- Ageing.

Course and treatment In these patients the prognosis is determined by the underlying condition. In patients with hyperfiltration injury there is a good rationale for using ACE inhibitors in the hope of preventing further renal damage; these agents reduce systemic and intraglomerular pressure, inhibit glomerular hypertrophy and decrease glomerular production of TGF-β, a cytokine which increases production of matrix proteins. They are certainly the anti-hypertensive agents of choice in most patients with hypertension and proteinuria: whether they should be used in normotensive patients is less certain.

Further reading

Meyrier A. Focal segmental glomerulosclerosis. To treat or not to treat? 2. Focal and segmental glomerulosclerosis is not a disease, but an untreatable lesion of unknown pathophysiology. Its treatment must not be uselessly hazardous. *Nephrology, Dialysis and Transplantation*, 1995; **10**: 2355–9.
Ponticelli C. Focal segmental glomerular sclerosis. To Treat or not to treat? 1. Is it worthwhile to give the adult patient with nephrotic syndrome the benefit of an adequate therapeutic trial? *Nephrology, Dialysis and Transplantation*, 1995; **10**: 2351–4.
Ritz E. Pathogenesis of 'idiopathic' nephrotic syndrome. *New England Journal of Medicine*, 1994; **330**: 61–2.

Related topics of interest

Disorders of extracellular volume (p. 54)
Minimal change glomerulonephritis (p. 121)
Reflux nephropathy (p. 154)
Renal biopsy (p. 163)
The kidney and hypertension (p. 202)

GLOMERULONEPHRITIS: GENERAL APPROACH

The term glomerulonephritis means inflammation of the glomeruli and related structures. The facts that the kidneys take 25% of the cardiac output and that the glomeruli are 'designed' to allow filtration of plasma mean that there is a very high flux of molecules, including immunoglobulins and foreign antigens, across the glomerular capillaries. Some of these molecules can cause inflammation in the basement membrane which supports the glomerular capillaries. The glomerular capillaries can also be involved by systemic vasculitis or by systemic insults causing endothelial damage, as in haemolytic uraemic syndrome or pre-eclampsia.

The classification of glomerulonephritis is confusing even to experts. Because the pathogenesis of many types of glomerulonephritis (GN) is not known, all pathologists can do is describe what is seen under the microscope. Unfortunately, there is a very poor correlation between clinical presentation and histological appearance: the same histological appearances may be seen in patients with asymptomatic urinary abnormalities, acute nephritic syndrome and nephrotic syndrome. However, certain patterns do emerge, as described below.

Light microscopy

There are only a few structures in the glomerulus, and they have a limited repertoire of responses to injury. Changes may either be 'diffuse', affecting all of the glomerulus, or 'segmental', affecting some part of the glomerulus but not others. 'Focal' changes affect some glomeruli and not others, although the fact that only a thin cross-section of each glomerulus is seen makes it hard to be sure that one is not missing segmental changes in apparently unaffected glomeruli.

1. Mesangial cells. These may proliferate ('mesangial proliferative GN'). Alternatively, macrophages, lymphocytes and polymorphs may infiltrate into the mesangium, causing similar appearances, as in 'diffuse proliferative GN'. Rarely, mesangial cells may be reduced in number after an acute insult ('mesangiolysis').

2. Mesangial matrix. This is secreted by mesangial cells. Increased amounts of mesangial matrix may be secreted in response to deposition of immune complexes or as a result of increased local expression of cytokines which alter the balance between production and degradation of matrix, as in diabetic glomerulosclerosis.

3. Glomerular capillaries. These may undergo necrosis, with fibrin deposition, as in some types of systemic vasculitis ('necrotizing GN').

4. Basement membrane. This may become thickened as a result of immune complex formation ('membranous GN') or split as a result of invasion by mesangial cells ('mesangiocapillary GN', also called 'membranoproliferative GN'); or may be congenitally thin ('thin basement membrane nephropathy').

5. Bowman's capsule. This may rupture as a result of severe glomerular inflammation or may show 'crescent' formation – proliferating cells adherent to the capsule which may later be replaced by fibrous tissue.

Other changes

Tubular atrophy and interstitial fibrosis are commonly seen in glomerulonephritis, and give better information on prognosis than the glomerular changes. However, these changes are non-specific.

Immune reactants

In addition to conventional stains, the presence of complement and immunoglobulins may be detected with the use of immunofluorescence or immunoperoxidase techniques.

Electron microscopy

Immune deposits may be identified clearly within the basement membrane or mesangium as electron-dense deposits. Some effacement or fusion of epithelial foot processes is seen in all proteinuric states, but is much more marked in minimal change GN than in other conditions.

Clinical presentation

- Asymptomatic haematuria or proteinuria.
- Acute nephritic syndrome.

- Nephrotic syndrome.
- Chronic renal failure.

Investigation

Accurate diagnosis of glomerulonephritis requires renal biopsy. There are no blood tests available for the diagnosis of primary glomerulonephritis.

- Serum creatinine, albumin, full blood count, viscosity.
- 24 h urine for creatinine clearance, protein excretion.
- Antineutrophil cytoplasmic antibodies (ANCA) are nearly always present in Wegener's granulomatosis and microscopic polyarteritis.
- Antinuclear antibodies and antibodies to double-stranded DNA are usually present in lupus nephritis.
- Low C3 and C4 complement occur variably in SLE, post-infectious GN, mesangiocapillary GN and cryoglobulinaemia. Congenitally low C4 is associated with an increased risk of SLE.

Management

Specific treatment of glomerulonephritis requires renal biopsy. Whatever the exact type of glomerulonephritis, tight control of hypertension reduces the risk of progressive renal damage.

Further reading

Mason PD, Pusey CD. Glomerulonephritis: diagnosis and treatment. *British Medical Journal*, 1994; **309**: 1557–63.

Related topics of interest

HAEMATURIA

Blood in the urine can appear as a result of disease anywhere from the glomerulus to the tip of the urethra. A few red cells are found in normal urine, but a pathological cause can nearly always be found for haematuria sufficient to be detected on dipstick testing or routine microscopy. However, microscopic haematuria is very common, and exhaustive investigation is not always justified.

Detection

1. Macroscopic haematuria. This is obvious, but can be confused with severe haemoglobinuria or myoglobinuria or with beeturia (caused by ingestion of beetroot).

2. Dipstick testing. This is widely used in screening. Positive tests are caused by haematuria (detection limit 5 cells/µl), haemoglobinuria, and myoglobinuria. False positives may be caused by iodine contamination of the sample container; positive dipstick tests for haematuria with negative microscopy are more usually due to false negative microscopy.

3. Bright field microscopy. This is the technique used in most microbiology labs, where detection of pyuria is the priority. Negative results may occur as a result of spontaneous lysis of red cells or by failure to detect 'ghost' forms.

4. Phase contrast microscopy. This is more time consuming but more sensitive for the detection of low-grade haematuria and also allows, in expert hands, differentiation of glomerular and non-glomerular haematuria and the detection of casts. Fresh specimens must be examined to avoid false negatives.

Causes

1. Urological malignancy. Including renal adenocarcinomas; urothelial tumours of the collecting systems, ureters, bladder, and urethra; prostate cancer; and penile carcinoma.

2. *Urothelial inflammation.* Caused by infection, stones or hypercalciuria (causing crystalluria).

3. *Polycystic kidney disease.*

4. *Necrosis of renal tissue.* As in papillary necrosis and renal embolism.

5. *Anticoagulation.* Investigation of patients who develop macroscopic haematuria on anticoagulants frequently shows a 'urological' cause. Over-anticoagulation may cause microscopic haematuria in the absence of disease.

6. *Glomerulonephritis.* Haematuria usually occurs with active inflammation of glomeruli but may occur with membranous nephropathy and minimal change disease. Absence of proteinuria does not exclude glomerulonephritis. Recurrent macroscopic haematuria shortly after the onset of upper respiratory infection is highly suggestive of IgA nephropathy or mesangiocapillary glomerulonephritis.

7. *Renal vein thrombosis.* This should be considered in patients with nephrotic syndrome who develop haematuria with or without flank pain.

8. *Alport's syndrome.*

9. *Thin basement membrane nephropathy.* This is an inherited disease characterized by abnormally thin basement membranes, detection of which requires careful analysis of electron microscope images. Haematuria may be microscopic or macroscopic and may be intermittent. The long-term prognosis is thought to be good; it is also called 'benign familial haematuria', but cases of renal failure have been described.

10. Loin pain haematuria syndrome. This comprises severe loin pain, flank tenderness and haematuria. It is much rarer in males than females. An increased tendency to vascular spasm after contrast injection during renal angiography suggests that this may be a form of 'renal migraine'. Deposition of C3 in arterioles is frequently present, but is non-specific. Abnormal illness behaviour is common, probably as a result of frustration with ineffective medical management. No satisfactory treatment exists, but autotransplantation and other surgical treatments have been tried.

11. Sickle-cell disease and trait. These can cause recurrent macroscopic haematuria due to sickling in the renal medulla.

12. Severe exercise. (Even if non-traumatic.)

13. Schistosomiasis. Involving the urothelium.

14. Factitious.

Investigation

Whether a 'urological' cause is sought before or after a 'nephrological' cause depends on age and on whether there are clues in the history, family history or initial investigation to one or other category of disease. As a general rule, urothelial malignancy is uncommon under the age of 40.

1. Culture of urine and urethral swab. This is required to exclude urinary tract infection, although this is a rare cause of asymptomatic haematuria.

2. Urine cytology. This should be performed in all patients at risk of malignancy, but negative results should not deter further investigation.

3. Phase contrast microscopy or automated cell size analysis. This may help to distinguish glomerular and non-glomerular bleeding and can be used to decide the direction of further investigations.

4. *Testing for proteinuria.* Proteinuria strongly suggests a renal cause of haematuria.

5. *Renal function.* This should be checked: renal impairment suggests either parenchymal renal disease or bilateral obstruction.

6. *Intravenous urography.* This is widely used as first-line investigation for upper urinary tract abnormalities, including stones and tumours.

7. *Ultrasonography.* This may be a useful alternative to urography but does not allow reliable detection of ureteric tumours or stones.

8. *Flexible cystoscopy.* This may be performed as an outpatient procedure to look for bladder tumours.

9. *Renal biopsy.* This is required for definitive diagnosis of parenchymal renal disease and shows glomerular abnormalities in at least 50% of patients with isolated microscopic haematuria (i.e. without hypertension, proteinuria, renal impairment, or symptoms). Biopsy should be performed if the results will alter management (seldom the case in the absence of proteinuria or renal impairment), if the prognosis needs to be known (e.g. for insurance purposes), or if a positive diagnosis is necessary to obviate the need for repeated urological investigations. An alternative is to assume that the patient has chronic glomerulonephritis and to arrange regular (usually annual) checks of blood pressure and renal function, with reassessment if either becomes abnormal.

Further reading

Arm JP, Peile EB, Rainford DJ, Strike PW, Tettmar RE. Significance of dipstick haematuria. 1. Correlation with microscopy of the urine. *British Journal of Urology*, 1986; **58**: 211–17.

Nieuwhof C, Doorenbos C, Grave W, *et al.* A prospective study of the natural history of idiopathic non–proteinuric hematuria. *Kidney International*, 1996; **49**: 222–5.

Topham PS, Harper SJ, Furness PN, Harris KPG, Walls J, Feehally J. Glomerular disease as a cause of isolated microscopic haematuria. *Quarterly Journal of Medicine*, 1994; **87**: 329–35.

Weisberg LS, Bloom PB, Simmons RL, Viner ED. Loin pain haematuria syndrome. *American Journal of Nephrology*, 1993; **13**: 229–37.

Related topics of interest

Glomerulonephritis: general approach (p. 81)
Imaging of the urinary tract (p. 110)
Proteinuria (p. 144)
Renal biopsy (p. 163)
Urinalysis and urine microscopy (p. 215)

HAEMODIALYSIS

Haemodialysis (HD) is the most widely and extensively used modality for the treatment of acute renal failure (ARF) and endstage renal failure (ESRF).

Technical aspects

Safe and effective HD can only be delivered if certain technical features are in place.

- Patients on HD are exposed to large amounts of water (used to prepare the dialysate). This needs to be rendered free of toxins (especially aluminium and chloramines), bacteria and endotoxins.
- Dialysate solutions may contain acetate or bicarbonate as the buffer base. Acetate solutions are less well tolerated by certain patients and are gradually being phased out of use, especially for acute HD.
- The dialyser shell is a tube or box containing four ports. Two ports communicate with the blood compartment and two with the dialysate compartment. These compartments are formed by multiple hollow fibres or multiple flat plates. Blood and dialysate flow in opposite directions separated by the dialysis membrane.
- The dialysis membrane may be made from cellulose, substituted cellulose, cellulosynthetic substances or synthetic materials (polysulphone, polyacrilonitrile, polyamide, polymethyl-methacrylate). These membranes differ in terms of permeability to different solutes, hydraulic permeability and complement activation.
- Dialysis machines consist of a blood pump, dialysate delivery system and a range of safety features to monitor the integrity of the extracorporeal circuit, prevent air embolism and maintain a standard dialysate concentration. Modern machines have optional and pro-grammable features to allow more individualized patient therapy.
- Secure long-term access to the circulation is best achieved by a forearm autologous radio-cephalic

arteriovenous fistula (Brescia–Cimino fistula).
When the venous limb of the access has
arterialized, it can be repeatedly cannulated and
blood removed/returned at rates of 200–500
ml/min. In patients with unsuitable venous
anatomy, alternative sites may be chosen,
synthetic grafts may be inserted or long-term
cuffed catheters placed in the central venous
system.
- Anticoagulation is achieved using systemic
unfractionated heparin administration, either by
bolus or infusion. In patients at high risk of
haemorrhage, epoprostenol (a prostacyclin
analogue) may be administered or regional hep-
arinization with protamine used.

Mechanisms of solute transport

- Solute removal is principally by diffusion down a
concentration gradient across a semi-permeable
membrane. Solute is also removed by convection,
if net ultrafiltration of fluid occurs during
treatment. Diffusive clearance depends upon
blood flow and dialysate flow rates, dialyser
surface area and the permeability of its
membrane to the solute. Ultrafiltration depends
upon the hydrostatic pressure across the
membrane and its hydraulic permeability.
- The clearance of specific molecules depends
upon their size, charge, volume of distribution
and degree of protein binding. Molecules and
drugs with a high volume of distribution are not
well cleared. In general, smaller solutes are better
removed than larger ones, which are better
cleared by convection.

Indications

- HD is indicated in ESRF, and is the mainstay of
RRT programmes. Within reason, practically any
patient can be treated with HD provided that
access to the circulation is available.
- Acute HD is indicated in the treatment of ARF
when a patient is compromised by, or is about to
be compromised by, severe hyperkalaemia,
acidosis, pulmonary oedema or uraemic
pericarditis. In addition, severe uraemia may

require therapy, even in the unlikely absence of these complications.

- In multi-organ failure, haemofiltration techniques are being increasingly applied in place of HD.

Prescription

- HD is delivered thrice weekly for the majority of patients. The number of hours of therapy depends upon the intensity of the available technology. With high blood-flow rates, high dialysate flow rates and large, very permeable dialysers the unit can deliver a high-efficiency HD treament in as little as 2 h. With less efficient technology, treatments of 4–5 h may be needed. All treatments should aim to deliver minimum targets of urea clearance. This is expressed as the normalized urea clearance parameter, Kt/V. For individual treatments a Kt/V of 1.2–1.4 should be sought.
- HD should control ECF volume and blood pressure. Compliance with fluid and salt restriction by the patient complements the removal of these during the treatment.
- Intradialytic morbid events such as cramp and hypotension can be avoided by changes in dialysate composition, avoidance of acetate as a buffer, use of ultrafiltration control and profiling sodium and water removal. In acute HD, rapid removal of urea during the first dialysis may lead to a shift of water into the brain with an acute cerebral disequilibrium syndrome.

Dialysis-associated amyloidosis (DAA)

- A variety of arthropathies and enthesopathies are described in long-term HD patients. Many of these are due to peri-articular deposition of a unique form of amyloid caused by polymerization of β_2-microglobulin. With increasing time spent on dialysis, progressive disabling problems may develop.
- β_2-microglobulin (molecular weight 11 800 Da) comprises the constant light chain of class I HLA antigens. It is normally filtered by the glomerulus, absorbed and catabolized by proximal tubular cells.

- Carpal tunnel syndrome and scapulo-humeral peri-arthritis (presenting with a stiff, painful shoulder) are the earliest clinical manifestations of DAA. After 10 years on dialysis, more than 50% of patients will have had such symptoms. Surgical release of the carpal tunnel syndrome is frequently necessary.
- A more diffuse and symmetrical large joint polyarthropathy is also well described. Significant visceral deposition of amyloid is unusual.
- DAA is now the most common cause of pathological fracture in dialysis patients. Fractures of the femoral neck are the most characteristic of these. Because the fractures occur across sites of amyloid deposition, primary non-union is common.
- Certain dialysis membranes exhibit better clearance of β_2-microglobulin than others. Similarly, membranes differ in their potential to excite an inflammatory response in the patient. There is some evidence to suggest that use of high-flux biocompatible synthetic dialysers from the beginning of RRT may be associated with a lower incidence of DAA-related problems.

Survival and outcome

- ESRF patient survival reflects co-morbid disease rather than modality-specific factors, although there is evidence of better survival with higher levels of urea clearance.
- The principal cause of death is cardiovascular disease, but sepsis is not infrequent and there is an increased relative risk of neoplasia.
- Inadequate nutrition may cause deceptively 'good' pre-dialysis blood urea and creatinine concentrations but is associated with poor outcome.

Further reading

Daugirdas JT and Ing TS (eds) *Handbook of Dialysis,* 2nd Edn. Boston: Little Brown and Company, 1994.

Related topics of interest

HAEMOFILTRATION

There is increasing application of haemofiltration techniques in the treatment of acute renal failure (ARF) and endstage renal failure (ESRF). Haemofiltration achieves solute removal by convection, rather than by diffusion (which is the principal mechanism of solute removal in haemodialysis).

Physiological principles and technology

- An artificial membrane (haemofilter) with a high hydraulic permeability is used to remove fluid from the circulating plasma volume at rates of 500–5000 ml/h. Simultaneous infusion of a pharmaceutically pure and physiologically balanced replacement fluid is servo-linked to the removal of filtrate.
- Net ultrafiltration is achieved by removing slightly more fluid than is replaced. Total filtrate produced depends upon the area and material of the haemofilter and the transmembrane hydrostatic gradient.
- Convective removal of solutes occurs with this technique. The total solute removal depends upon the total volume of filtrate produced, the concentration of solute in the plasma and the sieving coefficient of the membrane (a measure of the 'resistance' to solute movement with water).
- Replacement fluids contain sodium, calcium, magnesium, and chloride in concentrations similar to plasma. Lactate is usually used as the buffer, in place of bicarbonate. Variable concentrations of glucose are used, and the potassium concentration is generally adjusted for individual patients.
- Simple systems, consisting of a set of blood lines, a haemofilter, filtrate lines and replacement fluid lines are used with continuous arteriovenous haemofiltration (CAVH). More elaborate integrated systems, with safety features similar to haemodialysis machines, pump-driven blood flow and servo-controlled matching of filtrate and replacement fluid volumes are now widely available.

- Additional solute clearance by diffusion may be achieved by adding a dialysis limb to the system. The technique is then referred to as haemodiafiltration.

Applications

- In patients with multi-organ failure, standard haemodialysis (HD) may not be well tolerated, especially if there is a requirement to remove large volumes of fluid each day. In these circumstances, slow continuous haemofiltration techniques are often used. Their advantages have not been confirmed by controlled clinical trials.
- In slightly more stable patients recovering from ARF, there are concerns that HD can give rise to new lesions of ATN or cause changes in intra-cerebral pressure. Intermittent haemofiltration may be chosen for these patients. In some units 'unstable' chronic patients are treated by regular intermittent haemofiltration.
- Haemofiltration has better clearance of larger solutes than HD. Haemodialysis is more efficient at clearing small solutes. To achieve the highest level of clearance, a combined therapy called haemodiafiltration is used, which combines both modalities.

Haemodynamic stability

- It is unclear why haemofiltration seems to be better tolerated than HD. The haemofilter membrane is less bio-incompatible than a standard HD membrane. The replacement fluid is pharmaceutically pure, unlike the water used to make dialysate which may contain residual toxins or lipopolysaccharides. Convective solute re-moval may cause less intercompartmental shifts than diffusive clearance.
- Modern HD techniques, especially those incorporating sodium and ultrafiltration profiling may be tolerated just as well as haemofiltration. However, they still will not remove larger solutes as well.

CVVH

- One of the most common forms of slow con-tinuous renal replacement therapy is continuous veno-venous haemofiltration (CVVH). A single dual-lumen venous catheter is used with either an integrated system or with a modified, nurse-supervised, dialysis machine monitor.

- Typically used with patients with multi-organ failure, requiring high ultrafiltration to allow parenteral nutrition to continue.
- Access is established with a temporary catheter in the central or femoral veins. Continuous anticoagulation is provided with unfractionated heparin, low molecular weight heparin or epoprostenol, as appropriate. Filtrate is removed at 1000–3000 ml/h, depending on the catabolic state of the patient. Urea clearances of 15–30 ml/min are thereby achieved. Net ultrafiltration is adjusted as required to maintain the target ECF volume status.
- Careful daily assessment of fluid balance is important. Daily measurement of electrolytes, divalent ions and acid–base status is required. Difficulties may arise in patients with hepatic failure who may not metabolize lactate well and become paradoxically acidotic.
- Other continuous techniques are continuous arteriovenous haemofiltration (CAVH), continuous arteriovenous haemodiafiltration (CAVHD) and slow continuous dialysis.

Disadvantages

- Although well tolerated, continuous techniques are much less efficient than intermittent therapies. The need for them to be continuous may limit patient mobilization and requires prolonged anticoagulation with the attendant risks.
- Haemofiltration in continuous and intermittent mode is much more costly than standard haemodialysis because of fluid and haemofilter costs.

Further reading

Daugirdas JT and Ing TS (eds) *Handbook of Dialysis*, 2nd Edn. Boston: Little, Brown and Company, 1994.

Ronco C. Continuous renal replacement therapies for the treatment of acute renal failure in intensive care patients. *Clinical Nephrology*, 1993; **40**: 187–98.

Related topics of interest

HAEMOLYTIC URAEMIC SYNDROME AND THROMBOTIC THROMBOCYTOPENIC PURPURA

Haemolytic uraemic syndrome/thrombotic thrombocytopenic purpura (HUS/TTP) describes a spectrum of clinical syndromes in which there is thrombocytopenia, a microangiopathic haemolytic anaemia and ARF.

Classification

- HUS and TTP represent different clinical patterns of a pathophysiological continuum with considerable overlap.
- In HUS, renal problems tend to dominate.
- In TTP, haematological and neurological features are more marked.
- The epidemic form of HUS/TTP is the most frequent. Usually associated with bloody diarrhoea; 75–100% of cases follow infection by verocytotoxin-producing strains of *Escherichia coli*. The most frequently identified strain is 0157:H7. The exotoxins produced are designated VT1 and VT2 and are almost identical to the potent shiga toxin produced by *Shigella dysenteriae*.
- An endemic or sporadic form occurs without associated diarrhoea. It may be precipitated by cyclosporin and mitomycin and has been reported in transplant recipients, in collagen vascular diseases and with malignancies. Associated with scleroderma and accelerated phase hypertension. Post-partum cases occur which may represent an extension of the vascular abnormalities associated with eclamptic syndromes.
- Familial and relapsing cases are occasionally reported.

Epidemiology

- The most common cause of ARF in children, with an equal sex incidence.
- Shows seasonal variation, being more common in the warmer months.
- More common in those under 5 years.

- Shows a female preponderance in adults.
- Especially common in Latin American countries such as Argentina.

Clinical presentation

- Prodrome of watery and bloody diarrhoea. Abdominal pain may be intense with haemorrhagic colitis.
- Onset of renal and haematological problems is usually after 6–10 days, by which time the diarrhoea may have resolved.
- Oliguric ARF with microscopic haematuria and proteinuria. Occasionally non-oliguric ARF and macroscopic haematuria.
- Hypertension is unusual in diarrhoea-associated HUS/TTP.
- Hypertension is often severe in endemic/sporadic HUS/TTP.
- Skin petechiae and purpura are more common at the TTP end of the spectrum.
- Significant CNS disease may occur, with restlessness, disordered consciousness, ataxia and seizures.
- Endemic/sporadic cases tend to have a more insidious onset.

Pathophysiology

- Verocytotoxins (VTs) bind to a specific glycolipid receptor in the kidney and on the vascular endothelium – globotriasoyl ceramide-3 (GB3). This receptor is similar to the P1 blood group antigen to which VTs may also bind. Binding to the kidney depends upon the amount of GB3 receptor expressed. As this is more marked at the extremes of age, infants and the elderly are characteristically more frequently affected than older children and younger adults.
- Severe endothelial injury occurs. Platelets are consumed at this site and there is increased platelet activation. There is failure of vascular prostacyclin synthesis and abnormalities of von Willebrand factor (vWF) production and function have been described.
- Thrombosis and necrosis of intra-renal vessels may occur in the absence of cellular

inflammation. In the diarrhoea-associated form, there is predominantly glomerular capillary thrombosis. With the other forms, a pre-glomerular pathology with intimal proliferation of arterioles and small arteries is more common.

Laboratory features

- Thrombocytopenia is universal at some point in the illness.
- It is unusual for this to be severe enough to cause bleeding.
- Anaemia is common and often severe. Peripheral blood films show fragmented and deformed cells. There is an associated rise in LDH, unconjugated bilirubin and reticulocytes.
- Coomb's test is negative. Red cell enzymes and osmotic fragility are normal. Fibrin degradation products (FDP) are raised, but fibrinogen consumption is minor compared with platelet consumption. Disseminated intravascular coagulation (DIC) is unusual and prothrombin time normal – a coagulopathy suggests sepsis rather than HUS/TTP.
- Neutrophil leucocytosis may be quite marked; it is a marker of adverse prognosis.
- Patients are often hyponatraemic at presentation. Plasma urate, urea and creatinine are raised.

Management

- Diarrhoea-associated HUS/TTP generally resolves spontaneously over several days, so the mainstay of therapy is supportive. This may include red cell concentrate transfusion and dialysis.
- Controversy exists as to the utility of a variety of specific therapies used, most of which fail to exhibit the same benefits in controlled studies as in case series. Fresh frozen plasma has been administered, especially in adults. This is postulated to provide prostacyclin stimulating factor, vWF degrading factor, fibronectin and an inhibitor of platelet aggregating factors. It is frequently combined with plasma exchange. Infusion of prostacyclin has been advocated, as has administration of large doses of vitamin E.

Prognosis

- The natural history of diarrhoea-associated HUS/TTP is of spontaneous recovery, albeit with the potential for residual renal and neurological damage. Subsequent CRF develops in a number of survivors, possibly because of hyperfiltration and hypertension. Seventy per cent of affected children recover completely with no long-term sequelae.
- In those with endemic, sporadic, familial or other non-diarrhoea-associated illness the short-term and long-term prognoses are more guarded.

Further reading

Neild G. Haemolytic-uraemic syndrome. In: Cameron JS, Davison AM, Grünfeld J-P, Kerr D, Ritz E (eds) *Oxford Textbook of Clinical Nephrology*. Oxford: Oxford University Press, 1992; 1041–59.

Remuzzi G. HUS and TTP: variable expression of a single entity. *Kidney International*, 1987; **32**: 292–308.

Related topic of interest

Acute renal failure: general approach (p. 11)

HEPATO-RENAL SYNDROME

Hepato-renal syndrome (HRS) is a relatively specific pathophysiological entity occurring in patients with underlying liver failure. ARF may occur in jaundiced patients for a variety of other reasons. It is important to distinguish these, as the prognosis for the patient and the appropriate management are quite different.

Pathophysiology

- Occurs in patients with pre-existing chronic liver disease.
- Can occur with fulminant hepatic failure and with liver transplants undergoing rejection.
- Patients usually have a history of oedema, ascites, hyponatraemia, prolonged prothrombin time or variceal haemorrhage.
- Various abnormalities have been described. The GFR is commonly lower than predicted on the basis of plasma creatinine. There is a marked decrease in renal plasma flow, probably with a significant redistribution of regional intra-renal blood flow.
- Sympathetic nervous system activity is increased and increased circulating levels of cate-cholamines, ADH and angiotensin have been described. Failure to clear a circulating 'hepatopressin' has been postulated.
- The decrease in GFR is functional in nature. Renal biopsy shows no abnormality. Renal function is restored by successful liver transplantation. Kidneys with HRS will function normally if transplanted into a patient with normal hepatic function.

Presentation

- Rapidly progressive oligo-anuric ARF in a patient with already established significant liver disease.
- ECF volume is normal or increased. Usually there is no history of hypotension or sepsis and no recent exposure to nephrotoxic agents.
- Recent over-vigorous diuresis may be a precipitant.

- The urinary sediment is inactive. There is marked hyponatriuria.
- It is unusual for recovery to occur unless the patient receives a successful liver transplant. With very aggressive supportive care a few patients may survive for sufficiently long to recover renal function if there has been a spontaneous improvement in hepatic function.

Investigations

- Should focus on a vigorous search for alternative causes of ARF. ATN in these patients carries a prospect of renal recovery with good supportive management. HRS carries an essentially terminal prognosis unless liver transplantation is planned.
- Renal biopsy is seldom possible because of coagulation problems.

Management

- If liver transplantation is planned then meticulous supportive care is needed to maintain good fluid balance status, maintain nutrition, avoid bleeding and avoid cerebral oedema. This will usually necessitate ITU facilities.
- If renal replacement therapy is required, current practice favours the use of a continuous low-efficiency technique such as continuous veno-venous haemofiltration (CVVH).
- HRS may not recover for several days after liver transplantation. Persistence of ARF beyond 5–7 days suggests that an alternative cause of ARF has supervened.
- If liver transplantation is not planned and another cause for ARF unlikely, careful consideration of the possible futility of aggressive supportive care (especially renal replacement therapy) should promote discussion as to the ethics of continued therapy.

Further reading

Epstein M, Perez D, Oster JR. Management of renal complications of liver disease. *Journal of Intensive Care Medicine,* 1987; **3**: 71–86.

Sweny P. The hepatorenal syndrome. In: Rainford D, Sweny P (eds) *Acute Renal Failure*. London: Farrand Press, 1990; 83–112.

Related topics of interest

Acute renal failure: acute tubular necrosis and selected syndromes (p. 7)
Acute renal failure: general approach (p. 11)

IgA AND IgM GLOMERULONEPHRITIS

IgA nephropathy (also known as Berger's disease, not to be confused with Buerger's disease) is one of the most common types of chronic glomerulonephritis. Henoch–Schönlein purpura may be complicated by glomerulonephritis in which, like classical IgA nephropathy, there is mesangial deposition of IgA. These diseases have much in common and are best seen as part of a spectrum, particularly because Henoch–Schönlein glomerulonephritis may occur without the typical rash.

IgM nephropathy is much less well defined but shares many features with IgA disease.

IgA nephropathy

Presenting features
- Dipstick-positive haematuria and/or proteinuria.
- Recurrent macroscopic haematuria within 1–2 days of onset of upper respiratory tract infections.
- Recurrent macroscopic haematuria after exercise.
- Hypertension – IgA disease is a common cause of accelerated hypertension.
- Acute renal failure.
- Chronic renal failure.
- Nephrotic syndrome.

Associated diseases
- Liver disease – mesangial IgA deposition is common but seldom produces significant renal disease.
- Coeliac disease and dermatitis herpetiformis.
- Ankylosing spondylitis.
- Inflammatory bowel disease.

Diagnosis
Serum IgA may be raised but this is not diagnostic. IgA-class autoantibodies and circulating IgA–fibronectin complexes have been described, but none can be relied on for diagnosis.

Renal biopsy (by definition) shows deposition of IgA in the mesangium, with or without other immunoreactants (IgG, IgM, complement C3); a variety of histological patterns may be seen, the most common being an increase in mesangial cells and matrix, which may be focal and segmental or diffuse.

Natural history

Up to 30% of patients eventually progress to renal failure, although this figure may be artificially weighted by the inclusion of more patients with severe forms of the disease, as many patients destined to have a benign course (such as those with isolated microscopic haematuria) do not undergo renal biopsy and may not be included in long-term series. Complete remission (with disappearance of IgA deposits) is rare. A progressive course is predicted by the presence of hypertension, proteinuria, renal impairment and, on renal biopsy, sclerotic changes in glomeruli, interstitial fibrosis and tubular atrophy.

Pathogenesis

The IgA deposited in the glomeruli is primarily polymeric IgA1 and is derived from bone marrow plasma cells rather than gut-associated lymphoid tissue. Abnormal configurations of the carbohydrate hinge region of the IgA molecule are found and may cause the IgA to be deposited in the glomerulus and excite an inflammatory response. Numerous perturbations in cytokine and cellular control of IgA production have been described.

Management

Studies of treatment in IgA disease are complicated by the variable natural history.

1. Steroids. Several trials of steroid treatment have been reported, none showing unequivocal evidence of benefit. Reduction in proteinuria has been reported in controlled trials.

2. Steroids plus cytotoxic agents. Uncontrolled studies have claimed that steroids and azathioprine or cyclophosphamide improve outcome, but have yet to be confirmed by controlled studies. In the absence of firm evidence, it is reasonable to reserve this type of treatment for patients with a rapidly progressive course or those presenting with acute nephritic syndrome.

3. Phenytoin. Phenytoin reduces serum IgA levels but has no effect on progressive renal disease.

4. Control of hypertension. Because it would be unethical to leave hypertension untreated, controlled trials to confirm that antihypertensive treatment slows progressive renal disease have not been performed. However, all the evidence suggests a beneficial effect of tight blood pressure control. ACE enzyme inhibitors reduce proteinuria more than equipotent doses of other antihypertensives and are often used preferentially in proteinuric patients with IgA disease.

5. Fish oil. A randomized, controlled trial in patients with primary IgA disease and proteinuria (>1 g/day) showed a significantly slower rise in serum creatinine and significantly fewer patients dying or developing endstage renal failure in the treated group compared to a group receiving placebo. Unusually, there was no effect on proteinuria. Fish oil is thought to work by altering the secondary inflammatory response to glomerular disease, rather than attacking the root cause.

Henoch–Schönlein nephritis

Presenting features

Henoch–Schönlein purpura is a systemic leucocytoclastic vasculitis involving the skin, joints, intestines and kidneys. The purpuric rash affecting extensor surfaces predominantly on the legs is usually diagnostic, although other small vessel vasculitides can cause a similar appearance. The spectrum of clinical presentation of the renal lesion is similar to that of IgA disease.

Renal histology

Focal segmental glomerulonephritis with IgA deposition is the most common pattern. Crescents are seen in severe cases and indicate a poorer prognosis.

Natural history

In children, Henoch–Schönlein purpura and the associated renal disease are often self-limiting. In adults the course may be more prolonged, and progressive renal failure may occur.

Management	No treatment is of proven benefit. It is reasonable to consider a trial of steroids and azathioprine or cyclophosphamide in adults with crescents, severe proteinuria and impaired renal function, particularly if known to be of recent onset.

IgM nephropathy

The frequency with which IgM deposition is detected in kidney biopsies varies widely from series to series. IgM deposition may be non-specific, reflecting 'trapping' in areas of sclerosis. However, IgM is also seen in non-sclerosed glomeruli in association with a spectrum of renal disease similar to that seen with IgA deposition.

Minimal change with IgM	In some patients presenting with nephrotic syndrome, renal biopsy appearances are consistent with minimal change disease apart from the presence of IgM deposits. These patients may respond to steroids, but the response is often incomplete, and the prognosis poorer than in classical minimal change disease.
Mesangial proliferation with IgM	Proliferation of mesangial cells and increased mesangial matrix, as in IgA disease, is commonly seen in association with IgM deposition. Over 30% of these patients eventually develop renal failure. There is no treatment of proven benefit.

Further reading

Donadio JV. A controlled trial of fish oil in IgA nephropathy. *New England Journal of Medicine*, 1994; **331**: 1194–9.

Gwyn Williams D. IgA nephropathy. The commonest form of glomerulonephritis in industrialised countries. *British Medical Journal*, 1994; **308**: 74–5.

O'Donoghue DJ, Lawler W, Hunt LP, Acheson EJ, Mallick NP. IgM-associated primary diffuse mesangial proliferative glomerulonephritis: natural history and prognostic indicators. *Quarterly Journal of Medicine*, 1991; **79**: 333–50.

Peh CA, Clarkson AR. Treatment of IgA nephropathy. *Nephrology, Dialysis and Transplantation*, 1995; **10**: 1119–21.

Related topics of interest

Acute renal failure: general approach (p. 11)
Glomerulonephritis: general approach (p. 81)
Minimal change glomerulonephritis (p. 121)
Renal biopsy (p. 163)

IMAGING OF THE URINARY TRACT

As with any investigation, the first question is – what question is being asked, and how will the answer affect present or future management? Many of the investigations described here are expensive, and some involve significant exposure to ionizing radiation. In addition, contrast media may be nephrotoxic. Also, there is marked local variation in expertise and in the availability of some of the investigations described.

Ultrasound

Ultrasound is non-invasive, relatively cheap and widely available. Ultrasound is useful for assessment of renal size and for the detection of hydronephrosis and cysts, but less reliable for detection of cortical scars and stones. Abnormalities of the calyces and pelvis cannot be detected reliably using ultrasound.

Pulsed-wave Doppler imaging of the main renal artery shows characteristic wave-forms in renal artery stenosis. This method is time-consuming and observer-dependent, although very good results have been obtained in some centres.

Duplex ultrasound has also been used to assess intrarenal blood flow. The ratio of systolic to diastolic velocity within intrarenal arterioles is increased in conditions which cause renal swelling, such as acute rejection of a kidney transplant. This technique is of most use when repeated scans are obtained in the same patient.

Plain radiography

Radiography of the abdomen (KUB, kidneys, ureter and bladder) is a useful adjunct to ultrasound and allows detection of radio-opaque stones and of renal calcification (for instance, in renal tuberculosis and in nephrocalcinosis).

Intravenous urography

This remains the investigation of choice for the detection of stones (particularly if radiolucent); of chronic pyelonephritis, diagnosis of which requires the combination of cortical scars and underlying calyceal deformity; and of papillary necrosis. Drawbacks include contrast nephropathy and allergic reactions to contrast. The quality of images depends on renal function and, even with high doses of contrast, it is difficult to obtain adequate detail in the presence of significant renal impairment.

DMSA scanning

[^{99m}Tc]DMSA is taken up by functioning renal tubules. DMSA scanning is sensitive in the detection of focal parenchymal scars, for instance in children with reflux nephropathy or in adults with renal embolism.

DTPA and MAG3 scanning

[^{99m}Tc]DTPA is excreted largely by glomerular filtration and [^{99m}Tc]MAG3 by a combination of glomerular filtration and tubular secretion. Dynamic scanning can therefore give useful information on the relative contribution of the two kidneys to overall excretory function.

1. Captopril renography. This involves dynamic scanning before and after administration of 25 mg captopril. In the presence of renal artery stenosis, captopril results in greatly decreased glomerular filtration rate on the affected side, leading to a delay in uptake and subsequent excretion of isotope.

2. Diuretic renography. This is used to diagnose functionally important obstruction, and is particularly useful in distinguishing obstruction from post-obstructive dilatation of a collecting system. Dynamic scanning is performed during a diuresis, induced by a loop diuretic (usually frusemide). Delayed emptying during the excretion phase suggests obstruction.

CT scanning

CT scans are useful in the evaluation of renal cysts and solid masses and radiolucent stones. Contrast CT scans show characteristic appearances in acute pyelonephritis, but the importance of these findings is uncertain. Characteristic findings have been described in analgesic nephropathy.

MRI scanning

The use of this modality is rapidly evolving, and availability varies greatly, at least in the UK. Magnetic resonance imaging (MRI) is useful in the differential diagnosis of solid renal masses and cysts and in the staging of patients with renal malignancies. Magnetic resonance angiography may soon become the preferred alternative to conventional angiography in the diagnosis of renal artery stenosis.

Angiography   Renal angiography is invasive, requiring puncture usually of the femoral artery, but can be performed as a day-case procedure in most large hospitals. Detailed images not only of the main renal vessels but also of the intrarenal circulation may be obtained. This is the procedure of choice for the diagnosis of renal artery stenosis, intrarenal arteriovenous malformations and polyarteritis nodosa. In renal artery disease, angioplasty and/or stent insertion may be considered, particularly in fibromuscular disease.

Further reading

Cattell WR, Webb JAW, Hilson AJW. *Clinical Renal Imaging*. Chichester: John Wiley and Sons, 1989.

Related topics of interest

Analgesic nephropathy (p. 21)
Autosomal dominant polycystic kidney disease (p. 26)
Obstructive nephropathy (p. 125)
Reflux nephropathy (p. 154)
Urolithiasis (p. 235)

INTERSTITIAL NEPHRITIS

Interstitial inflammation and fibrosis are commonly seen in a wide variety of renal diseases. Progressive renal failure is associated not only with glomerulosclerosis but also with tubular atrophy and interstitial fibrosis; in fact the degree of tubular atrophy is a better predictor of prognosis in glomerulonephritis than the degree of glomerular inflammation. However, in some cases the interstitial inflammation is the primary event.

Acute interstitial nephritis

Presentation

Acute interstitial nephritis is responsible for up to 15% of cases of acute renal failure. Hypertension and oliguria are unusual, and polyuria can occur. Often there are no specific features and the disease will not be recognized unless the possibility is actively considered.

- Proteinuria is usually mild and comprises low molecular weight 'tubular' proteins.
- Microscopic haematuria is common, but red cell casts are rare.
- White cells (including eosinophils, detection of which requires staining) and white cell casts are seen.
- There may be evidence of tubular dysfunction, including renal tubular acidosis, aminoaciduria, glycosuria and impaired sodium conservation and urinary concentrating ability.

Allergic interstitial nephritis may cause more specific symptoms in addition, including:

- fever,
- eosinophilia (and eosinophiluria),
- rash.

Infection

Many infections can incite an inflammatory response within the renal interstitium, including:

- Streptococci, diphtheria, *Brucella, Legionella* and other bacterial pathogens.
- Tuberculosis.

- Spirochaetes: syphilis and *Leptospira*.
- Viruses, including BK virus, measles, Epstein–Barr, cytomegalovirus and Hantaviruses.

In addition, ascending urinary infection can cause primary bacterial interstitial nephritis, particularly in poorly controlled diabetes; here there is active proliferation of organisms within the renal parenchyma, which may progress to abscess formation.

Drug allergy

The list of drugs which have been reported to cause interstitial nephritis is so long that the only sensible policy is to suspect drug-induced interstitial nephritis in any patient who develops acute renal failure following ingestion of any drug. Drugs for which this is a relatively common reaction (often those which also cause drug rashes) include:

- Penicillins, particularly methicillin.
- Cephalosporins.
- Sulphonamides.
- Rifampicin.
- Non-steroidal anti-inflammatory drugs (which can also cause a number of other renal diseases).
- Diuretics, particularly thiazides.
- Phenytoin.
- Allopurinol.
- Omeprazole.

Herbal medicines

Recently a rapidly progressive fibrosing interstitial nephritis was described in young women taking a Chinese herbal slimming medicine containing chopped magnolia blossoms. Some mushrooms can cause a similar picture.

Treatment

Treatment is usually that of the underlying cause. In immunologically mediated interstitial nephritis there is sometimes a dramatic apparent response to steroids, with resolution of fever and rapid improvement of renal function, but controlled trials have not been done and spontaneous recovery usually occurs. Whether steroids help to prevent chronic interstitial fibrosis after the acute insult is unknown.

Chronic interstitial nephritis

Drug–induced renal disease is dealt with elsewhere (see p. 57).

Toxic

- Chronic lead intoxication, usually a result of occupational exposure, can cause hypertension, gout and a chronic non-specific tubulointerstitial nephritis which may cause progressive renal failure.
- Chronic cadmium intoxication may also cause chronic tubulointerstitial damage, with tubular proteinuria, evidence of proximal tubular dysfunction and osteomalacia due to renal calcium wasting. Progressive renal failure may occur.
- Balkan nephropathy is a slowly progressive interstitial nephritis found in families living in Balkan villages, with a highly restricted geographical distribution. Patients have an increased risk of urothelial tumours. The most likely cause appears to be a plant toxin contaminating wheat, combined with genetic susceptibility.

Sarcoidosis

Sarcoidosis may cause a granulomatous interstitial nephritis, which usually responds to steroid treatment but may leave irreversible renal damage. Sarcoidosis has also been associated with a variety of types of glomerulonephritis.

Nephrocalcinosis

Deposition of calcium-containing crystals in the interstitium may occur in chronic hypercalcaemia, renal tubular acidosis, and in hyperoxaluria.

Sjögren's syndrome

Occasionally, the T-cell-mediated inflammation of lacrimal and salivary ducts in this condition also affects renal tubular cells, causing type 1 (distal) renal tubular acidosis with hypokalaemia. Significant renal impairment is less common. Renal biopsy shows a lymphocytic interstitial nephritis.

Further reading

Cameron JS. Allergic interstitial nephritis: clinical features and pathogenesis. *Quarterly Journal of Medicine*, 1988; **66**: 97–115.

Jones CL, Eddy AA. Tubulointerstitial nephritis. *Pediatric Nephrology*, 1992; **6**: 572–86.

Nolan CR, Anger MS, Kelleher SP. Eosinophiluria: a new method of detection and definition of the clinical spectrum. *New England Journal of Medicine*, 1986; **315**: 1516–19.

Related topics of interest

Acute renal failure: general approach (p. 11)
Drug-induced renal disease (p. 57)
Renal involvement in connective tissue diseases (p. 171)
Renal tubular acidosis (p. 191)
Viral diseases and the kidney (p. 235)

MEMBRANOUS NEPHROPATHY

Membranous nephropathy is the most common cause of nephrotic syndrome in adults. It may be primary, or secondary to a wide range of systemic diseases. The pathogenesis is unknown and treatment controversial.

Presenting features

Eighty per cent of patients present with nephrotic syndrome, the remainder with lesser degrees of proteinuria. Up to 50% of patients are hypertensive at presentation. Occasional patients may present with acute renal failure as a complication of nephrotic syndrome.

Associated diseases

In 20–30% of patients, membranous nephropathy appears to be secondary to an underlying disease:

- Infection – hepatitis B, malaria, schistosomiasis, many others.
- Malignancy – carcinomas in many sites, lymphomas (particularly Hodgkin's), leukaemias. The malignancy may be occult when the patient first presents.
- Autoimmune diseases – SLE and variants, Hashimoto's thyroiditis, myasthenia gravis, many others.
- Sarcoidosis.
- Drugs and toxins – gold, penicillamine, captopril.

Complications

Renal vein thrombosis occurs in up to 50% if carefully looked for, and there is an increased risk of deep venous thrombosis elsewhere. The risk of cardiovascular disease is increased in patients with persistent nephrotic syndrome.

Investigations

- 24 h urine for protein, creatinine clearance.
- Tests for protein selectivity show an unselective pattern but are not often performed.
- FBC, biochemical screen, viscosity.
- Serum cholesterol.
- Hepatitis B surface antigen.
- ANA, dsDNA, ENA, thyroid antibodies.
- Chest radiography; consider other investigations for underlying malignancy.

- Cross-linked fibrin degradation products (? renal vein thrombosis).
- Renal biopsy.

Natural history

The clinical course is unpredictable. Sustained remission may occur after years of nephrotic-range proteinuria. Renal function may start to decline and then improve, or, more commonly, there may be inexorable progression to endstage renal failure once renal function has started to decline. Renal failure may eventually develop in 15–20%. Persistent nephrotic syndrome causes profound muscle wasting and malaise. The prognosis for patients with malignancy-associated disease is poorer than for those with similar malignancies without the nephrotic syndrome. The risk of recurrence of the disease in a renal transplant is around 10%, but it may also occur *de novo*.

Pathology

Renal biopsy shows thickening of the glomerular basement membrane, which forms 'spikes' and, later, 'chains' around the deposits. There is usually little or no inflammatory response to the deposits. Tubular and vascular lesions indicate a worse prognosis. Staining for immune reactants shows diffuse granular IgG and C3 with or without other reactants: a 'full house' of staining for IgG, IgA, IgM, C3, C4 and C1q is seen in SLE. Electron microscopy shows subepithelial dense deposits.

Pathogenesis

In experimental animals, membranous nephropathy can be produced by induction of an autoantibody against an antigen present on the tubular brush border and on glomerular epithelial cells. However, despite an extensive search, the equivalent autoantigen in humans has not been identified.

Carriage of the HLA-DR3 antigen is associated with increased susceptibility to the disease.

In tumour-associated membranous nephropathy there is evidence for deposition of antigen–antibody complexes in which the antigen is derived from the tumour.

Management

1. *General.* Oedema may be treated with loop diuretics, taking care to avoid hypovolaemia, which could cause worsening of renal function. Hypertension should be treated, aiming for a blood pressure less than 140/90 mmHg.

2. *Diet.* A high-protein diet does not improve serum albumin or muscle bulk but does increase urinary protein losses. Dietary protein intake should not exceed 1 g/kg ideal body weight. Sodium restriction may help to control oedema and potentiates the antiproteinuric effect of ACE inhibitors.

3. *Anticoagulants.* These should be used in patients with persistent nephrotic syndrome unless there are strong contraindications.

4. *Angiotensin-converting enzyme inhibitors.* These reduce protein excretion independent of the cause, and can lessen morbidity from the nephrotic syndrome. Whether reduction of proteinuria improves subsequent outcome in this situation is not yet known.

5. *Lipid-lowering therapy.* This should be considered in persistently nephrotic patients.

6. *Steroids and cytotoxic therapy.* Steroids alone may hasten remission but do not prevent renal impairment. Controlled trials have shown that combinations of steroids with chlorambucil induce remission and reduce loss of renal function. However, since many patients are destined to go into spontaneous remission, this regimen is not widely used. An alternative is to reserve treatment for those patients whose renal function shows progressive deterioration. Uncontrolled studies suggest that cytotoxic treatment may stabilize or improve renal function in this situation.

7. *Cyclosporin.* This has also been shown recently to be effective in reducing proteinuria and rate of loss of renal function in patients with membranous nephropathy and deteriorating renal function.

Further reading

Cattran DC, Greenwood C, Ritchie S, *et al.* A controlled trial of cyclosporine in patients with progressive membranous nephropathy. *Kidney International,* 1995; **47**: 1130–5.

Hebert LA. Therapy of membranous nephropathy: what to do after the after (meta) analyses. *Journal of the American Society of Nephrology,* 1995; **5**: 1543–5.

Pauker SG, Kopelman RI. Hunting for the cause: how far to go. *New England Journal of Medicine,* 1993; **328**: 1621–4.

Remuzzi G, Bertani T, Schiepatti A. Grand round: idiopathic membranous nephropathy. *Lancet,* 1993; **342**: 1277–80.

Related topics of interest

Complications of the nephrotic syndrome (p. 35)
Glomerulonephritis: general approach (p. 81)
Renal biopsy (p. 163)

MINIMAL CHANGE GLOMERULONEPHRITIS

Minimal change glomerulonephritis is the most common cause of nephrotic syndrome in children but can occur at any age. In most patients, no cause is found. Although it is clearly an immunologically mediated disorder, it is related to abnormal T-cell function rather than immune complex deposition. A lymphocyte-derived factor which increases glomerular permeability would explain many of the features of the disease, but this factor has not been definitively identified.

Synonyms
- Minimal change nephropathy.
- Minimal change disease.
- Lipoid nephrosis.
- Idiopathic nephrotic syndrome (also includes focal segmental glomerulosclerosis).

Presenting features
Patients usually present with full-blown nephrotic syndrome. Careful monitoring with urine dipsticks of patients with a previous episode can allow detection of a relapse before the onset of severe proteinuria and oedema, but this stage usually progresses to full-blown nephrotic syndrome unless treated.

Hypertension and/or microscopic haematuria occur in 20–30% of patients.

Renal impairment, and even acute renal failure, may occur.

A history of atopic disease is commonly present.

Causes
- Usually 'idiopathic' (unknown).
- Mercury, lead.
- Hodgkin's disease, other malignancies.
- Drugs: NSAIDs (often associated with a mild interstitial nephritis); sulphasalazine and derivatives; others.
- Food allergy.
- Infectious mononucleosis, HIV infection.

Investigations
1. Protein selectivity. The proteinuria in nephrotic syndrome is usually highly selective for albumin and transferrin rather than larger protein molecules. Measurement of the ratio of clearance of transferrin to IgG (by paired measurements in serum and urine)

allows the estimation of selectivity. Unselective proteinuria makes minimal change disease very unlikely.

2. 24 h urine. For protein and creatinine clearance.

3. Renal biopsy. This is the only way of confirming the diagnosis. However, it is not usually necessary to confirm the diagnosis in children unless there are atypical features, such as non-selective proteinuria or poor response to treatment.

Pathology

No abnormality of glomeruli can be seen on light microscopy or on staining for immune reactants – hence the name 'minimal change'. 'Foam cells' (lipid-laden tubular cells) may be prominent (hence 'lipoid nephrosis') but may occur in other causes of severe nephrotic syndrome. On electron microscopy, the normal tentacle-like 'foot processes' of epithelial cells along the basement membrane are fused ('effaced') into a continuous layer. Foot process effacement is not unique to minimal change disease, but is usually more complete than in other causes of proteinuria.

Complications

- Hypercoagulable state (urinary loss of anticoagulant proteins) causing increased risk of deep-vein thrombosis (DVT) and renal vein thrombosis.
- Hypercholesterolaemia.
- Impaired immunity (urinary loss of immunoglobulins).
- Severe oedema, ascites, pleural effusions.

Natural history

Spontaneous remission can occur, but it is seldom justified to leave a patient untreated in case this happens, as persistent nephrotic syndrome carries a significant mortality. Following induction of remission, at least 90% of children will relapse if followed for long enough, but the risk of relapse decreases with time. Relapses often appear to be precipitated by minor upper respiratory infections.

Treatment

1. Supportive. Diuretics help to clear oedema but may cause or worsen hypovolaemia. In children with evidence of hypovolaemia, 20% human albumin solution is recommended but can precipitate acute pulmonary oedema if over-used. Prophylactic subcutaneous heparin may be considered but long-term anticoagulation should not be necessary because the underlying condition can be corrected. Prophylactic penicillin should be considered in patients with ascites, who are at risk of spontaneous pneumococcal peritonitis.

2. Corticosteroids. These are the mainstay of treatment. Children should be treated with prednisolone 60 mg/m^2/day (max. 80 mg) for 4 weeks, then 40 mg/m^2/day for 4 weeks, followed by a tapering dose over 4 weeks. Remission of proteinuria and diuresis are usually seen within the first few weeks. Low-dose and abbreviated regimens carry a higher risk of early relapse. Adults respond more slowly, and should be treated with 1 mg/kg/day for 8–12 weeks, followed by 0.5 mg/kg/day for a further 6–8 weeks and then by a tapering dose over 8 weeks.

3. Cyclosporin. This has also proved useful in maintaining remission, and may be considered as a steroid-sparing agent in patients with frequent relapses. Most patients relapse when the drug is withdrawn. Dangers of long-term use include induction of hypertension and chronic cyclosporin nephrotoxicity.

4. Cyclophosphamide. This is the only drug known to reduce the risk of subsequent relapses. Because of its toxicity, it should only be offered to patients with frequent relapses. A dose of 2–3 mg/kg/day, with regular monitoring of the white blood cell count, is introduced once the patient is in remission, and continued for 12 weeks (maximum cumulative dose 200–250 mg/kg). With this regimen the risks of infertility, bladder toxicity, and secondary malignancy are low.

5. *Levamisole.* In contrast to the other agents used, this is an immunostimulant. In children with steroid-dependent, frequently relapsing nephrotic syndrome it has been shown to be effective in maintaining remission for up to 100 days. It has not been studied in adults.

Further reading

British Association for Paediatric Nephrology. Levamisole for corticosteroid–dependent nephrotic syndrome in childhood. *Lancet,* 1991; **337**: 1555–7.

Korbet SM. Management of idiopathic nephrosis in adults, including steroid–resistant nephrosis. *Current Opinion in Nephrology and Hypertension,* 1995; **4**: 169–76.

Niaudet P, Habib R. Cyclosporine in the treatment of idiopathic nephrosis. *Journal of the American Society of Nephrology,* 1994; **5**: 1049–56.

Related topics of interest

OBSTRUCTIVE NEPHROPATHY

Partial obstruction in the urinary tract is an important cause of renal failure. The longer obstruction is present, the less recovery of renal function can be expected after relief of obstruction. Early recognition is therefore vital.

Apart from the unusual situation of complete bilateral obstruction, urine volume and flow rate are **normal** in obstructive renal disease, and indeed some patients may be polyuric. Because serum creatinine does not rise above the upper limit of normal until the glomerular filtration rate has halved, complete unilateral obstruction will not necessarily be detected by measurements of serum creatinine.

Causes

Obstruction can occur at any point from the collecting systems to the urethral orifice. Listed below are some of the more common causes.

1. Prostatic bladder outflow obstruction. This is one of the major causes of renal failure in men over the age of 50, and frequently presents late. Most, but not all, patients have had the typical lower urinary tract symptoms of hesitancy, urgency, and frequency for years before detection of renal failure.

2. Prostatic malignancy. This can also cause bladder outflow obstruction but may also cause bilateral obstruction where the ureters enter the bladder.

3. Bladder cancer. This usually presents with macroscopic haematuria but may occasionally present with renal failure due to bilateral ureteric obstruction.

4. Retroperitoneal fibrosis. RPF causes bilateral ureteric obstruction, usually at the level of the mid-ureter. It is caused by an autoimmune response to an insoluble lipid, ceroid, leaking from a diseased aorta and occurs in association with aortic atherosclerosis or in association with an inflammatory aortic aneurysm. It is therefore predominantly a disease of patients over the age of 50. Malaise, non-specific aching back pain, and low-grade fever are common, and there is usually an acute phase response.

5. *Stones.* Stones seldom cause renal failure unless they are causing bilateral obstruction, blockage is present in a single functioning kidney, or there is associated nephrocalcinosis as in primary hyperoxaluria. Obstruction by a staghorn calculus is, however, an important cause of unilateral loss of renal function.

6. *Pelvi-ureteric junction (PUJ) obstruction.* This is caused by a fibrous band, which may be congenital or acquired, at the junction of the pelvis and ureter. Flank pain during diuresis is highly suggestive, but the condition may be asymptomatic until a grossly hydronephrotic kidney is discovered incidentally.

7. *Congenital.* Congenital causes include posterior urethral valves in boys.

8. *Neurogenic bladder.*

Pathophysiology

Increased pressure in the upper urinary tract leads to a reflex shut-down in renal blood flow and glomerular filtration; to infiltration of macrophages and other inflammatory cells; and eventually to tubular dilatation and atrophy with surrounding interstitial fibrosis. Hypertension and oedema are rare unless obstruction is complete and bilateral, and some patients may be frankly volume-depleted as a result of impaired water and sodium conservation. Urinalysis is unremarkable.

The obstructed kidney is particularly susceptible to ascending infection, which in the presence of obstruction can cause severe parenchymal scarring.

Post-obstructive diuresis

Relief of obstruction results in a gradual return of glomerular filtration but, if obstruction has been bilateral, may be complicated by severe polyuria and sodium wasting, resulting in severe hypovolaemia (and pre-renal renal failure) unless corrected by intravenous fluid replacement. This requires intensive medical management; it soon becomes difficult to be sure that the polyuria is not being 'driven' by the continued fluid replacement.

Diagnosis

1. Ultrasound scanning. This is the mainstay of diagnosis: a dilated collecting system ('hydronephrosis') and ureter ('hydroureter') are strongly suggestive of obstruction. However, these appearances may persist after relief of obstruction (the 'baggy pelvis') and do not confirm current obstruction. Obstruction may also occur without dilatation, particularly if there is peri-renal fibrosis as a result of infection (e.g. tuberculosis) or malignancy.

2. Intravenous urography. This may also show hydronephrosis and, if renal function is adequate, is better for imaging of the ureters to determine the site of obstruction. However, as with ultrasound, it is difficult to distinguish current from previous obstruction.

3. Diuresis isotope renography using ^{99m}Tc MAG3. This is the non-invasive investigation of choice for the diagnosis of current obstruction, which causes delayed washout of isotope from the pelvis during diuresis.

4. Invasive investigation. This may sometimes be necessary to confirm the nature and site of obstruction. Retrograde pyelography allows detailed imaging of the collecting systems even in severe renal failure. Antegrade pyelography requires introduction of a percutaneous nephrostomy tube, but allows measurement of the pressures generated by infusion of fluid into the renal pelvis ('Whitaker test'), the seldom-used 'gold standard' for the diagnosis of obstruction.

Treatment

Relief of obstruction is necessary to restore renal function. Clearly, the risks of attempted relief of obstruction have to be weighed against the risks of loss of renal function, and this will depend on the general condition of the patient and on whether or not obstruction is bilateral.

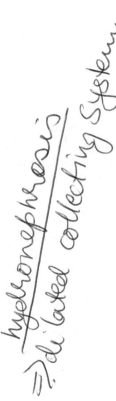

hydronephrosis

2) dilated collecting system

1. Percutaneous nephrostomy tubes. These allow direct drainage of an obstructed kidney and may 'buy time' for a more definitive procedure but are suitable in the short term only.

2. Internal stents. These may be inserted antegradely or retrogradely between the renal pelvis and the bladder to relieve ureteric obstruction. Because of the danger of encrustation and infection, these have to be changed every 6–12 weeks. They are of most use in the medium-term management of obstruction while the patient is prepared for definitive surgery.

3. Surgical procedures. These may include prostatectomy, pyelolysis (for PUJ obstruction), ureterolysis, open and percutaneous removal of stones, and construction of an ileal conduit in the case of inoperable bladder disease.

4. Extracorporeal shock-wave lithotripsy. This is an increasingly effective option for many stones.

5. Steroids. These cause resolution of retroperitoneal fibrosis and may be used as an adjunct to surgical 'ureterolysis' or in combination with internal stents. The response is monitored by measurement of acute-phase response (e.g. ESR, CRP) and by serial CT scanning of the retroperitoneal mass.

Further reading

Klahr S. Obstructive uropathy. In: Greenberg A (ed.) *Primer on Kidney Diseases.* London: Academic Press, 1994; 184–9.
O'Reilly PH. Diuresis renography: recent advances and recommended protocols. *British Journal of Urology*, 1992; **69**: 113–20.
Webb JAW. Ultrasonography in the diagnosis of renal obstruction. *British Medical Journal*, 1990; **301**: 944–6.

Related topics of interest

OTHER INHERITED CAUSES OF RENAL DISEASE

A wide range of inherited conditions can affect the kidney. Recent advances in molecular biology and genetics have added considerably to the understanding of many of these conditions.

Alport's syndrome

- Onset in childhood with haematuria, high-tone deafness and glomerular disease progressing to ESRF in late teens or early adult years. Ophthalmic abnormalities are also seen, including lenticonus and perimacular flecks. Macrothrombocytopenia and leiomyomatosis are less frequent associations. Males are more frequently and severely affected than females. The incidence is about 1 in 5000 live births. Anti-GBM disease is occasionally seen in transplanted patients.

- Pathognomic biopsy feature is irregular thickening and 'basket-weave' splitting of the basement membrane on electron microscopy.

- Caused by different mutations in the genes controlling the expression of type IV collagen in the basement membrane. Six α-chains of type IV collagen exist. Genes coding for each of these have been identified. The α1 (IV) and α2(IV) chains are coded by the *COL4A1* and *COL4A2* genes respectively. These are found on chromosome 13. *COL4A3* and *COL4A4* genes, found on chromosome 2, code for a3(IV) and a4(IV) chains. *COL4A5* and *COL4A6* genes code for a5(IV) and a6(IV) chains and are found on the X chromosome.

- 80% of affected kindreds show X-linked dominant pattern of inheritance. In these kindreds a number of mutations of the *COL4A5* gene have been identified. In female carriers, random inactivation of the other (normal or abnormal) X-chromosome in somatic cells throughout the body leads to a variable clinical expression.

- Most of the remaining kindreds have an autosomal recessive inheritance with mutations of the COL4A3 gene on chromosome 2.

Nail-patella syndrome

- Also called oncho-osteodysplasia. Features include ungual hypoplasia/dysplasia and bony abnormalities such as iliac horns. Forty per cent of cases have renal disease, which may progress to ESRF.
- On electron microscopy the GBM is irregularly thickened. Collagen bundles are a characteristic feature.
- Autosomal dominant inheritance. Gene defect on chromosome 9.

Thin basement membrane disease

- Presents with microscopic haematuria, but with normal BP and normal renal function. Good long-term prognosis.
- Renal biopsy is normal on light microscopy but glomerular basement membrane is seen to be thin on EM.
- Autosomal dominant inheritance. Relevant gene(s) not identified.

Medullary cystic disease (MCD)

- Also referred to as juvenile nephronophthisis. Presents at the end of the first decade with polyuria, polydipsia, impaired urinary concentration and ultimately CRF.
- The autosomal recessive version occurs in 1 in 50 000 live births.
- Autosomal dominant inheritance with onset in adult life is also reported.

Von-Hippel Lindau syndrome

- Familial disorder with angiomatous or cystic lesions in the kidneys. Also retinal angiomas, cerebellar and spinal haemang ioblastomas and adrenal phaeochromocytomas. Increased risk of bilateral renal cell carcinoma. May be confused with autosomal dominant polycystic kidney disease.
- Autosomal dominant inheritance. Gene defect on chromosome 3.

Tuberous sclerosis	• Presents with hamartomas of skin, brain, eye, heart and kidney. Fifty per cent of patients are educationally subnormal. Most have seizures. Facial angiofibromas, hypopigmented macules and ungual fibromas are easily identified. Angiomyolipomas may occur in the kidney, as may renal cysts.
	• Gene linkage is heterogeneous. At least four loci have been identified. TSC1 locus is on chromosome 9, with chromosome 16 having the TSC2 locus. This occurs beside the gene for autosomal dominant polycystic kidney disease (ADPKD).
	• Autosomal dominant inheritance. Incidence of 1 in 20 000 live births.
Anderson–Fabry disease	• Lower abdominal angiokeratomata in a 'bathing suit' distribution, with intermittent painful crises. Peripheral neuropathies, cardiac dysrythmias and cardiac failure may occur. Proteinuria and CRF begin in the third decade, usually proceeding to ESRF by the fourth or fifth decade.
	• Deficiency of lysosomal enzyme α-galactosidase A.
	• X-linked inheritance. Female carriers occasionally express a milder phenotype.
Cystinosis	• Non-nephropathic and nephropathic forms. The most severe is the infantile nephropathic form with an incidence of 1 in 200 000 live births. Presents in first year of life with Fanconi's syndrome, acidosis, polyuria and growth retardation and ultimately progresses to ESRF.
	• Extra-renal features include progressive loss of vision, hypothyroidism and infiltration of CNS, muscle, liver and pancreas.
	• Diagnosis made by detecting corneal deposition on slit-lamp examination or by measuring cystine in leucocytes or macrophages.
	• Renal biopsy shows a 'swan-neck' deformity of proximal tubules, with cystine crystals deposited in glomerular, tubular and interstitial cells.

- Therapy with cysteamine or phosphocysteamine may delay progression. This disease recurs after organ transplantation.
- Autosomal recessive inheritance.

Cystinuria

- The most common genetic cause of urolithiasis in adults. Responsible for up to 5% of urinary tract stones in childhood.
- Defective amino acid transport in epithelia of kidney and intestine.
- Marked urinary losses of cystine (and other dibasic amino acids such as ornithine, arginine, lysine). Cystine has poor solubility and crystallizes easily, leading to stone formation, obstruction and CRF.
- Treatment is with high fluid intake, urinary alkalinization and, in resistant cases, D-penicillamine.
- Autosomal recessive inheritance.

Hyperoxaluria

- Two distinct biochemical entities, with similar clinical presentations.
- The most common variant is PH1 (primary hyperoxaluria type I). Presents with recurrent urinary calculi and hyperoxaluria, subsequently progressing to CRF and ESRF.
- Results from a defect in glyoxalate metabolism with overproduction of oxalate and glycolate. The hepatic enzyme alanine glyoxalate aminotransferase is deficient. A minority respond to therapy with vitamin B_6. Liver transplantation corrects the enzymatic defect.
- Autosomal recessive inheritance.

Congenital nephrogenic diabetes insipidus

- Arginine vasopressin acts on the V2 receptor on the collecting duct. This act of binding leads to insertion of the water-selective channel aquaporin-2 into the cell membrane.
- Two different defects have recently been identified. In one there is a mutation leading to an abnormality of the V2 receptor. In the other there is a defect in the structure of aquaporin-2.
- Both defects have X-linked inheritance pattern.

Further reading

Gilbert-Barness EF, Opitz JM, Barness LA. Hereditable malformations of the kidney and urinary tract. In: Spitzer A and Avner ED (eds) *Inheritance of Kidney and Urinary Tract Diseases*. Norwell MA: Kluwer Academic Publishers, 1990; 327–400.

Reeders ST. Molecular genetics of hereditary nephritis. *Kidney International,* 1992; **42**: 783–92

Related topics of interest

Autosomal dominant polycystic kidney disease (p. 26)
Urinary tract masses and cysts (p. 224)
Urolithiasis (p. 229)

PERITONEAL DIALYSIS

Increasing numbers (>100 000 worldwide) of ESRF patients are being treated by continuous ambulatory peritoneal dialysis (CAPD). Increasingly, automated peritoneal dialysis (APD) systems are also being applied. Despite considerable disadvantages in using peritoneal dialysis in the treatment of ARF, it continues to be employed in this role in certain centres.

Applied peritoneal physiology

- 1–3 l of sterile dialysate are infused into the peritoneal cavity via a catheter. This is left to dwell for between 1 and 8 h and subsequently drained. Being a low-efficiency system compared with HD, repeated exchanges are necessary on a more or less continuous basis.
- Solute removal is achieved by diffusion from blood into the dialysate. For a given solute, this depends upon effective peritoneal surface area, permeability of the membrane to the solute and the concentration gradient. After the fluid has been *in situ* for some time, the dialysate begins to equilibrate with the blood and the concentration gradient decreases.
- Water removal is achieved by establishing an osmotic gradient into the peritoneal cavity. This depends upon the osmotic agent used and the permeability of the peritoneal membrane to it. Water removal depends upon effective peritoneal surface area, hydraulic permeability of the membrane and the osmotic gradient. Glucose is the usual osmotic agent. After the fluid has been *in situ* for some time, the dialysate glucose diffuses into the patient, thereby dissipating some of the osmotic gradient.
- Solute removal also occurs by convection, travelling with water. The amount removed depends upon the net water flux, the concentration of the solute in the plasma and the sieving coefficient of the membrane (a measure of its resistance to a solute travelling with a solvent). Molecules such as albumin tend to move by convection rather than by diffusion.

Indications

- Treatment of ESRF, provided the patient is capable of self-care or has a carer to assist with exchanges. Relative contraindications are the presence of abdominal wall hernias, previous abdominal surgery, significant diverticular disease (increased risk of peritonitis) and large body size (total clearance achieved with PD may be insufficient to keep the patient well).
- Treatment of ARF when haemodialysis or haemofiltration facilities are not available. Being relatively inefficient, interfering with dia-phragmatic excursion and being prone to infectious complications makes PD unattractive in this role.

Prescription

- In CAPD, the objective is to control salt and water balance and uraemia. Usually 4 daily exchanges of 2.0–2.5 l volume are performed. Different concentrations of glucose provide a choice of osmotic gradients to match net ultrafiltration to the patient's needs.
- Small solute clearance can be directly measured and targets for this have been proposed. Normalized urea clearance is expressed as Kt/V. It is proposed that a Kt/V of 1.8–2.0 per week should be sought, with a creatinine clearance of 60 l/wk/1.73 m^2.
- Many CAPD patients have residual renal function. This makes an important contribution to their total weekly small solute clearance.
- Increasingly, the inability to achieve adequate small solute clearances in larger patients with no residual renal function and poor peritoneal permeability is leading to transfer to HD.

Peritonitis

- This remains a major problem. Intra-peritoneal antibiotics can be used to manage 80% of patients, many as outpatients. Infection rates of 1 per 20 patient-months are now standard. Peritonitis remains a major reason for drop-out to haemodialysis.
- Peritonitis may be due to a variety of organisms. In the past, coagulase-negative staphylococci

were the most common pathogens. These have
declined with improvements in training and in
connection systems, which diminish intra-luminal
contamination. *Staphylococcus aureus* is now
more common and is associated with persistent
nasal carriage. The proportion of cases due to
Gram-negative organisms has increased. These
may spread from the bowel. This may reflect the
higher prevalence of diverticular disease seen as
the PD population ages. Fungal peritonitis is
uncommon but severe and usually follows
protracted use of broad-spectrum antibiotics.

Exit-site infections (ESI)

- Although giving rise to more minor problems in
  terms of symptoms, exit-site infections can be
  protracted and are more predictive of catheter
  loss than peritonitis rates. The organism usually
  involved is *Staphylococcus aureus*. Nasal
  carriage is important, and eradication of this leads
  to decreased ESI rates.

Membrane permeability

- Each patient's peritoneal membrane is different.
  In particular, permeability to solutes differs. A
  high permeability to solutes leads to good solute
  clearance but poor ultrafiltration, as the osmotic
  gradient generated by glucose is rapidly
  dissipated by its diffusion into the patient. Low
  permeability allows excellent ultrafiltration, but
  poor solute clearance. A number of different
  osmotic agents are now available to address the
  problem of high permeability to glucose.
- Peritoneal transport characteristics may be
  defined with a peritoneal equilibration test (PET),
  which facilitates selection of the most rational
  CAPD regimen. Over time, many patients
  develop a more permeable peritoneum with
  consequent ultrafiltration failure.

Other problems

- Weight gain, often to obese levels, is frequently
  seen. Absorption of glucose (providing 200–700
  kcal/day) from dialysate is the principal cause.
  For similar reasons, dyslipidaemias (especially
  hypertriglyceridaemia) are more marked with PD

than in CRF or HD. Protein loss (often >5 g/day) may also contribute to dyslipidaenia.

- Abdominal wall hernias may develop or worsen during peritoneal dialysis. This occurs more frequently in CAPD than in APD, as intra-abdominal pressures are more raised when patients are sitting or standing than when supine. In some centres, meshes to strengthen the abdominal wall are placed at the time of catheter insertion.
- Dialysate may leak into the pleural space or subcutaneously.

APD

- Automated peritoneal dialysis is increasingly employed. More rapid cycles are performed on patients while they sleep; they then have either a dry day or fewer exchanges during the daytime.
- Patient choice and convenience is a major indication for APD. It is also much more suitable for patients with ultrafiltration failure due to a high peritoneal permeability. Intra-abdominal pressure effects are less marked during the recumbent period at night. APD has been used, with daytime exchanges to augment total daily small solute clearances, in patients not achieving targets on CAPD.

Survival and outcomes

- Patient survival, as on HD, is principally a reflection of co-morbid risk factors rather than modality-specific factors.
- Studies on patient survival on PD and HD have given conflicting results. Apart from in the United States, there is no evidence to suggest that patient survival differs between modalities.
- Similarly, there is no evidence to suggest that subsequent transplant function differs between modalities.
- There is no evidence to suggest that elderly patients, diabetics or patients with heart disease have a better outcome on CAPD.
- CAPD has a limited duration of use. Few patients remain on this modality for more than 10 years, in stark contrast to HD.

Further reading

Daugirdas JT and Ing TS (eds) *Handbook of Dialysis,* 2nd Edn. Boston: Little, Brown and Company, 1994.

Gokal R. Current state and future trends in peritoneal dialysis. *Proceedings of the Royal College of Physicians Edinburgh,* 1996; **26**: 402–7.

Related topics of interest

Chronic renal failure (p. 31)
Haemodialysis (p. 89)
Renal osteodystrophy (p. 180)

POST-INFECTIOUS AND MESANGIOCAPILLARY GLOMERULONEPHRITIS

Post-streptococcal glomerulonephritis

This is relatively rare, and certainly much rarer than IgA disease, with which it is often confused, as both may present after upper respiratory tract infection. Only certain 'nephritogenic' strains of streptococci are associated with glomerulonephritis, and for reasons which are unclear these strains have become less common over the past 20 years.

It is important to remember that streptococcal infections can also produce acute renal failure as a result of toxic shock syndrome causing acute tubular necrosis.

Presentation	The patient develops haematuria (macroscopic or microscopic), proteinuria, hypertension, oedema and oliguric renal impairment 10–20 days after an acute group A streptococcal infection (e.g. pharyngitis, impetigo or cellulitis).
Investigation	• Full blood count, creatinine, urea and electrolytes. • Urine: non-selective proteinuria, seldom in the nephrotic range. Microscopy shows red cell casts and dysmorphic red cells. • Throat swab may allow identification of the causative organism, although the infection may have cleared or been treated by the time of presentation. • Complement: very low C3, low C4: levels remain low for 6–8 weeks. • Rising titres of serum antibodies to streptococcal antigens (e.g. streptolysin O, DNAase B) provide evidence of recent streptococcal infection, and remain elevated for up to 6 months. Antistreptolysin O titres do not rise after skin infections.
Pathology	Renal biopsy shows diffuse proliferative glomerulonephritis, with polymorph infiltration and mesangial and endothelial cell proliferation.

Granular IgG and C3 are found in capillary loops, seen as electron-dense 'humps' projecting from the epithelial side of the basement membrane on electron microscopy.

Natural history
Spontaneous resolution of renal impairment and fluid retention within 2–4 weeks is usual. Dialysis is seldom required. Haematuria and proteinuria may persist for months but eventually disappear. The long-term prognosis is thought to be good, particularly in children, but some patients with adult onset of disease have subsequently developed endstage renal failure.

Treatment
Hypertension and fluid retention should be treated with loop diuretics. Severe hypertension with hypertensive left ventricular failure or encephalopathy may require dialysis and ultrafiltration. Neither antibiotics nor steroids have any effect on the natural history of the disease. Since recurrences are rare, prophylactic antibiotics are not justified.

Other post-infectious glomerulonephritides

Endocarditis
Endocarditis can cause renal damage both as a result of septic emboli and as a result of immune-complex-mediated glomerulonephritis. Chronic infection of ventriculo-atrial shunts also causes glomerulonephritis. In both cases, a mesangiocapillary pattern is found.

Staphylococcal
Acute renal failure occurring 1–2 weeks after the onset of staphylococcal infection may be due to post-staphylococcal glomerulonephritis. Hypertension is less common than in post-streptococcal disease, but the renal biopsy appearances are indistinguishable.

Mesangiocapillary glomerulonephritis

The term mesangiocapillary glomerulonephritis (MCGN) describes a group of immune-complex diseases with characteristic histological appearances which can be caused by a number of different diseases or may occur as a 'primary' disease. Clinical presentation is also varied. Membranoproliferative GN is an alternative term.

Pathology

There are three subtypes. In each, there is lobulation of the glomerulus, mesangial cell proliferation, increased mesangial matrix, and splitting or re-duplication of the basement membrane.

1. Type 1. Immunoglobulins and C3 are present in the mesangium and in the sub-endothelial part of the basement membrane.

2. Type 2. Linear deposition of C3 is present along the basement membranes. Electron microscopy shows dense deposits along the lamina densa of the basement membranes of glomeruli and also of tubules and arterioles. Ring-like complement deposits are also seen in the mesangium.

3. Type 3. This combines features of type 1 MCGN with those of membranous nephropathy.

Immunology

Evidence of ongoing complement consumption is often found. Type 1 disease involves activation of both classical and alternative pathways (usually by circulating immune complexes), resulting in low C3, C4 and C1q. Type 2 involves activation of the alternative pathway, resulting in normal C4 and C1q but low C3 levels. IgG autoantibodies which activate the alternative pathway are frequently found in type 2 disease: these are called 'C3 nephritic factor'.

Cryoglobulins should also be present.

Associations

Both type 1 and type 2 disease may be found in association with a variety of systemic diseases, for instance:

- SLE.
- Mixed essential cryoglobulinaemia.
- Cryglobulinaemia secondary to chronic infection, including hepatitis C.

- Chronic infections such as subacute bacterial endocarditis (SBE), HIV.
- Homozygous sickle-cell disease.
- Intravenous drug abuse.
- Partial lipodystrophy (possibly reflecting the involvement of the complement system in regulation of fat turnover).
- Malignancies.

Presentation

Type 1 MCGN usually presents with nephrotic syndrome, but may present with asymptomatic haematuria, proteinuria, hypertension or chronic renal impairment, or with acute nephritic syndrome. Slow progression to endstage renal failure is usual, and spontaneous remission is rare.

Type 2 MCGN often presents with acute nephritic syndrome or with macroscopic haematuria following upper respiratory infections (similar to IgA nephropathy).

Recurrence of MCGN in a transplanted kidney is more common than in patients with other forms of glomerulonephritis, but causes transplant failure only in a minority.

Treatment

An underlying cause should be searched for and treated where possible.

1. Non-specific. Hypertension should be controlled carefully. In proteinuric patients an ACE inhibitor should be considered.

2. Specific. In 'idiopathic' MCGN there is no evidence of benefit from steroids or cytotoxic agents. Two studies have shown stabilization of renal function with antiplatelet agents or anticoagulants, but with no effect on proteinuria, and there is a good case for a trial of aspirin in patients with MCGN and deteriorating renal function.

Further reading

Donadio JV, Offord KP. Reassessment of treatment results in membranoproliferative glomerulonephritis, with emphasis on life-table analysis. *American Journal of Kidney Diseases*, 1989; **14**: 445–51.

Nissenson AR, Baraff LJ, Fine RN, Knutson DW. Post-streptococcal glomerulonephritis: fact and controversy. *Annals of Internal Medicine*, 1979; **91**: 76–86.

Tejani A, Ingulli E. Post-streptococcal glomerulonephritis. Current clinical and pathological concepts. *Nephron*, 1990; **55**: 1–5.

Related topics of interest

PROTEINURIA

Detection of increased urinary protein excretion is of major prognostic importance in many different clinical situations. In primary renal disease it is highly predictive of progressive renal failure. Even in the absence of defined renal disease it is a powerful risk marker for cardiovascular disease. Detection of proteinuria should therefore raise two questions: is it due to treatable primary renal disease, and is there anything that can be done to reduce cardiovascular risk?

Terminology

- 'Microalbuminuria': increased excretion of albumin below the range normally detectable by standard dipsticks.
- 'Clinical proteinuria': detection of proteinuria using dipsticks. May also be called 'macroalbuminuria'.
- 'Selectivity ratio': ratio of clearance of large protein to smaller protein (e.g. IgG : transferrin).
- 'Nephrotic range proteinuria': excretion of greater than 3 g protein per 24 h.
- 'Tubular proteinuria': excretion of low molecular weight proteins normally reabsorbed by proximal tubules.
- 'Bence-Jones proteinuria': excretion of immunoglobulin light chains.

Detection

1. Dipstick testing. This is relatively insensitive to light chains and globulins. The detection limit is around 300 mg/l. False positives may occur in highly alkaline urine (the test strip uses a pH-sensitive dye buffered at pH 3.0, whose pH sensitivity is altered by proteins); false negatives may occur in dilute urine.

2. Precipitation methods. These are used in the laboratory for quantitation of protein excretion. Precipitation of protein by acids causes measurable increases in turbidity. Protein excretion is either expressed in g/24 h (requiring collection of a 24-h urine sample) or as protein : creatinine ratio (which can be measured on a random sample); the latter relies on the fact that creatinine excretion rate is relatively constant. Proteinuria of greater than 300 mg/24 h or 30 mg/mmol creatinine is pathological.

3. Electrophoresis. This allows qualitative assessment of which proteins are present, enabling detection of tubular proteins and polyclonal and monoclonal light chains.

4. Specific assays. Specific assays are available for albumin as well as a number of other urinary proteins and enzymes. Stick tests are now becoming available for detection of 'microalbuminuria' but are expensive, observer-dependent and do not allow for variations in urine concentration. Measurement either of 24-h albumin excretion, overnight albumin excretion or albumin:creatinine ratio give a more accurate assessment of the albumin excretion rate.

Causes

1. Functional. Increased protein excretion may occur as a result of fever, exercise and congestive cardiac failure. Upright posture also increases protein excretion, both in subjects with normal kidneys and in those with pathological proteinuria. Functional proteinuria is seldom greater than 1 g/24 h.

2. Glomerular disease. Proteinuria may be selective (suggesting minimal change disease) or non-selective and may vary in amount from microalbuminuria to massive proteinuria. Heavy proteinuria is predictive of progressive renal failure; some evidence suggests that this is because proteinuria itself causes tubular damage and interstitial scarring.

3. Tubular disease. Tubular damage leads to decreased reabsorption of low molecular weight proteins and, to a lesser extent, of albumin. Increased release of tubular enzymes such as N-acetyl-β-D-glucosaminidase from damaged cells may also contribute.

4. Overflow. Massively increased filtration of proteins may overwhelm the reabsorptive capacity of the tubules and 'spill over' into the urine. This occurs in light chain overproduction, resulting in Bence-Jones proteinuria. Other examples include lysozyme in acute leukaemia and amylase in acute pancreatitis.

Microalbuminuria

1. Diabetics. Microalbuminuria in a patient with diabetes is highly predictive both of increased cardiovascular mortality and of progression to clinical diabetic nephropathy. Early detection offers more opportunities for prevention of progression and for intervention to reduce cardiovascular risk. Screening of all diabetics at risk of nephropathy is therefore justified.

2. Non-diabetics. An increased frequency of microalbuminuria has been shown in several conditions, including essential hypertension and atherosclerosis, and predicts the presence of dyslipidaemia and other cardiovascular risk markers. It has not been shown to predict progressive renal disease in these conditions. Screening these groups for microalbuminuria is not justified as there is no evidence that antiproteinuric treatment alters the prognosis. Attention should be directed to treatable risk factors such as smoking, obesity and hyperlipidaemia.

Low-grade proteinuria

Clinical proteinuria is also highly predictive of cardiovascular mortality in the general population, and in the long term is also associated with an increased risk of hypertension and endstage renal disease. How far to investigate a patient with proteinuria in the range 0.3–2.0 g/24 h and no clues to the cause of proteinuria on history and examination is controversial. Postural proteinuria should be excluded by measuring protein (or albumin) excretion rate in urine collected after overnight recumbency; no further investigation is required if this is normal, as the long-term prognosis is very good. Renal biopsy is usually recommended only if there are other pointers to renal disease, such as renal impairment, hypertension or haematuria.

Myeloma should be excluded in patients over 40. Whether or not an underlying cause is found, attention should be paid to treatable cardiovascular risk factors.

High-grade proteinuria

Proteinuria of greater than 2 g/24 h usually indicates significant primary renal disease. Renal biopsy should be performed to look for treatable causes (e.g. SLE, membranous nephropathy, minimal change disease) and to enable prediction of prognosis.

Treatment

Treatment to reduce proteinuria may be justified in nephrotic syndrome but not in asymptomatic proteinuria.

1. Diet. Paradoxically, protein restriction reduces proteinuria, probably by reducing intraglomerular pressure. Restriction of dietary protein intake to 0.6 g/kg ideal body weight plus daily urine protein losses may be considered in nephrotic syndrome but requires careful dietetic monitoring to avoid negative protein balance and muscle catabolism. Conversely, high protein diets may be deleterious.

Dietary sodium restriction may be helpful in the management of severe fluid retention and potentiates the antiproteinuric effect of ACE inhibitors.

2. Angiotensin-converting enzyme inhibitors. These reduce intraglomerular pressure and glomerular permeability, and reduce proteinuria to a greater extent than other antihypertensive agents. This effect is most pronounced in combination with dietary sodium restriction.

3. Non-steroidal anti-inflammatory drugs. These also reduce proteinuria but often at the expense of reducing the glomerular filtration rate. Their role in nephrotic syndrome is uncertain.

Further reading

Beetham R, Cattell WR. Proteinuria: pathophysiology, significance and recommendations for measurement in clinical practice. *Annals of Clinical Biochemistry*, 1993; **30**: 425–34.

Iseki K, Iseki C, Ikeyima Y, Fukiyama K. Risk of developing end-stage renal disease in a cohort of mass screening. *Kidney International*, 1996; **49**: 800–5.

Related topics of interest

RAPIDLY PROGRESSIVE GLOMERULONEPHRITIS (RPGN)

Glomerular disease progressing rapidly to dialysis-requiring renal failure is a relatively unusual clinical occurrence. Any idiopathic glomerular disease can transform into RPGN, usually with an underlying morphology of crescentic GN. More usually, RPGN is a manifestation of one of a number of systemic vasculitides, particularly those affecting small vessels and associated with circulating antineutrophil cytoplasmic antibodies (ANCA).

Systemic vasculitides and ANCA-associated renal diseases

- Vasculitis is a non-specific response of blood vessels to infective or immunological insults. Focal or systemic vasculitic lesions are found in a wide range of multisystem autoimmune conditions. These include SLE, bacterial endocarditis, Henoch-Schönlein purpura, essential cryoglobulinaemia and rheumatoid arthritis.
- A group of conditions is recognized in which blood vessels appear to be the primary site of injury. Giant cell arteritis and Takayasu's arteritis affect larger vessels. Kawasaki's disease and classical polyarteritis nodosa (CPAN) affect medium-sized vessels. Smaller vessels are affected in Wegener's granulomatosis (WG), microscopic polyangiitis (MPA) and Churg-Strauss syndrome.
- ANCA are relatively uncommon in vasculitic syndromes in which circulating or deposited immune complexes are prominent (such as SLE and Henoch-Schönlein purpura). They are more likely to be found in the so-called 'pauci-immune' vasculitides and are strongly associated with WG, MPA and Churg-Strauss syndrome. Sixty to eighty per cent of patients with what was previously described as 'idiopathic pauci-immune RPGN' are now known to be ANCA positive.
- The incidence of these conditions is increasing to about 15 cases pmp per annum. Peak incidence is in the fifth and sixth decades of life, with a further peak in the elderly population.

Antineutrophil cytoplasmic antibodies (ANCA)

- ANCA may be detected by indirect immunofluorescence (IIF). Serum from affected patients is applied to ethanol-fixed normal neutrophils. Fixation of ANCA to these is detected using labelled antibodies to human immunoglobulins.
- Two patterns may be seen. A diffuce cytoplasmic pattern is termed c-ANCA and a perinuclear pattern is termed p-ANCA.
- The specific antigens to which ANCA are directed (in these diseases) are now identified, c-ANCA are directed against proteinase-3 and p-ANCA are directed against myeloperoxidase. Both antigens are components of neutrophil granules. More specific radio-immune assay (RIA) and enzyme-linked immunosorbent assays (ELISA) are now available to detect and measure the antibodies directed aganst these specific antigens.
- c-ANCA have a high sensitivity (>85%) and specificity (>90%) for active WG. p-ANCA are more associated with MPA and have somewhat lower sensitivity and specificity.
- ANCA have been directed in other conditions, such as inflammatory bowel disease, liver disease and Felty's syndrome. A broader specificity exists in these conditions, with neutrophil antigens such as elastase, lactoferrin, peroxidase and cathepsin G being the targets.

Presentation

- Prodromal symptoms of malaise, arthralgia, myalgia and weight loss are common. Skin rashes and episcleritis may have occurred.
- Pulmonary involvement occurs in up to 50% of cases. In Churg-Strauss syndrome, asthma with eosinophilia is a pathognomonic feature. In MPA, and especially in WG, pulmonary infiltrates, nodules and cavities may be detected. Pulmonary haemorrhage may occur.
- ENT involvement is most prominent in WG. This may cause nose pain, mucosal ulceration and destruction of nasal bones with saddle-nose deformity. Otitis media and loss of hearing may

occur. Sub-glottic stenosis is frequent but is rarely severely symptomatic.

- Vasculitis of the heart, liver, nervous system and GI tract also occurs.
- Renal disease usually presents as ARF with haematuria and proteinuria. There is often very severe renal failure which requires immediate dialysis. Renal biopsy characteristically shows a focal and segmental necrotizing glomerulonephritis with crescent formation. There may also be an extraglomerular vasculitis affecting smaller blood vessels. Granulomas may be detected in WG but not always, as the pathological changes are usually focal.

Investigations

- Usual investigations for glomerular disease and ARF. Ultrasonography will show normal-sized, non-obstructed kidneys.
- ANCA and anti-GBM antibodies should be sought. Ideally access to both IIF and ELISA assays should be available.
- Pulmonary function tests to measure lung volumes and transfer factor. Flow-loops will detect sub-glottic stenosis.
- Renal biopsy or biopsies of the skin, lung or nasal mucosa may be needed to make a tissue diagnosis.

Treatment

- Corticosteroids (e.g. prednisolone, 1 mg/kg/day orally) and cytotoxic agents (usually cyclophosphamide, 1-3 mg/kg/day orally) are the mainstay of therapy. Apart from in patients with severe pulmonary haemorrhage or in those presenting with dialysis-requiring renal failure, plasma exchange has not been shown to offer any specific advantage.
- Most patients will enter clinical remission with standard induction therapy. Up to 60% of dialysis-requiring patients will regain independent function. However, many of these will subsequently develop ESRF and return to dialysis.

- During maintenance therapy, azathioprine is often substituted for cyclophosphamide, to minimize long-term toxicity.
- Relapse occurs in 30–50% of patients. Long-term monitoring, even in those who are ANCA-negative and in clinical remission, is necessary. ANCA titres frequently rise before a clinical relapse. Proactively increasing immuno-suppression in this situation may decrease the total immunosuppression needed to control a relapse.
- Experimental therapies such as humanized monoclonal antibodies with anti-T-cell (anti-CD52 and anti-CD4) activity have been successfully used in resistant cases. Results with intravenous immunoglobulin therapy have been mixed. Co-trimoxazole may be useful in prevention of relapse, particularly in WG localized to the ENT.

Anti-GBM antibody disease

- Goodpasture's syndrome refers to any clinical situation in which there is both lung haemorrhage and glomerulonephritis. However, it is a term usually restricted to a disease in which autoantibodies are directed against the glomerular basement membrane (GBM) and the pulmonary basement membrane. These target organs are damaged by a type II immune reaction.
- Clinical presentation is classically with haemoptysis, severe renal impairment, normal-sized kidneys on ultrasonography and an active urinary sediment. In some cases the pulmonary involvement may be less marked. There is a suggestion that prodromal systemic symptoms are less marked than with the vasculitides.
- Renal biopsy shows a crescentic glom-erulonephritis with extensive glomerular necrosis. All glomeruli are usually affected to the same extent. On immunofluorescence there is linear staining for IgG along the GBM, often with co-localized complement (C3). Lung biopsy shows haemorrhage without substantial leucocytic infiltration.

- Circulating anti-GBM antibodies may be detected by ELISA or RIA techniques.
- The target antigen has been identified as the α-3 chain of Type IV collagen. Susceptibility to the disease may be linked with the MHC class II antigen, DRw2.
- Clinically detectable lung haemorrhage is found in 60–75% of cases. This can be confirmed by finding an increased transfer factor for carbon monoxide on pulmonary function testing. Pulmonary involvement is more severe in those who smoke.
- Therapy is with plasma exchange, corticosteroids and alkylating agents (usually cyclophosphamide). This is often life-saving if pulmonary haemorrhage is extensive, but it is unusual for patients presenting with dialysis-requiring renal failure to recover independent functions. Patients can be transplanted once the production of circulating autoantibodies has been stopped.
- A variant of anti-GBM disease has been reported on several occasions in patients with Alport's syndrome who receive a cadaveric renal transplant.

Further reading

Gaskin G and Pusey CD. Systemic vasculitis. In: Cameron JS, Davison AM, Grünfeld J-P, Kerr D, Ritz E (eds) *Oxford Texbook of Clinical Nephrology*. Oxford: Oxford University Press, 1992; 612–36.

Jennette JC and Falk RJ. Diagnosis and management of glomerulonephritis and vasculitis presenting as acute renal failure. *Medical Clinics of North America*, 1990; **74**: 893–908.

Turner N and Rees AJ. Antiglomerular basement membrane disease. In: Cameron JS, Davison AM, Grünfeld J-P, Kerr D, Ritz E (eds) *Oxford Textbook of Clinical Nephrology*. Oxford: Oxford University Press, 1992: 438–56.

Related topics of interest

REFLUX NEPHROPATHY

Vesico-ureteric reflux (VUR) is a common underlying abnormality in childhood UTI. In association with infection, VUR frequently leads to a chronic interstitial nephropathy which can manifest as hypertension and progressive CRF. Presentation is frequently delayed until adult life, especially in female patients.

Pathophysiology

- VUR may be secondary to bladder outflow obstruction or occur with a neurogenic bladder. It may also occur as a primary congenital defect at the vesico-ureteric junction.
- The severity of reflux may be graded with voiding cystourethrography. Grading is determined by the degree of reflux, the presence of dilatation of the ureter and pelvi-calyceal system and the presence of intra-renal reflux. Intra-renal reflux is more common at the poles of the kidney, because of the compound configuration of papillae at these sites. Associated abnormalities of the ureteric orifice ('stadium' and 'golf hole') are also used in grading severity.
- It is uncommon for urinary tract sepsis alone to cause a chronic interstitial nephropathy. Intra-renal reflux of infected urine with interstitial ischaemia and high intra-pelvic and intra-pelvi-calyceal pressures does damage the interstitium. Affected areas fibrose and scar. The first infection is especially important in this regard.
- Renal scarring is more likely with infection in infancy, infection by MS-fimbriate *E. coli*, higher grades of VUR, delayed treatment and concomitant obstruction. Progressive CRF reflects the interstitial nephropathy and is adversely affected by hypertension, recurrent symptomatic UTIs and pregnancy.

Prevalence

- VUR is found in 5–25% of young children with UTI. Reflux nephropathy is the most common cause of hypertension in childhood.

- Reflux nephropathy can lead to CRF, and up to 10 patients per million population per annum develop ESRF from this cause.
- There is an increased incidence of VUR in first-degree relatives of patients with reflux nephropathy. Screening will detect VUR in 15–30% of members of certain families.

Investigations

- Urine culture should be performed with the sampling technique appropriate to the patient's age group. Renal function should be assessed, blood pressure measured and proteinuria quantified.
- Ultrasonography should be performed early after a documented UTI in infants and children under the age of 5 years. This will demonstrate any existing scars or urinary tract dilatation. DMSA scanning is more sensitive, but transient defects may be seen just after infection. Persistence of these after a period of urine sterility is a more specific feature of renal scarring. Voiding cystourethrography should be performed if abnormalities are detected. Antibiotic prophylaxis should be given until after investigations are complete.
- In older children, voiding DTPA scans may be more easy to perform and assess. However, a similar sequence to the above should generally be followed.
- In adults with suspected reflux nephropathy, ultrasonography and intravenous excretion urography (IVU) are the investigations of choice. Loss of renal substance, focal scarring at the renal poles and dilated pelvi-calyceal systems with clubbing are characteristic. VUR may no longer be present in the mature urinary tract.

Management

- It is not yet clear whether any therapy prevents long-term renal impairment in kidneys damaged at the time of presentation. As a result, early treatment of UTI in infants and younger children, with rapid performance of diagnostic tests, is most important.

- In children under 2 years of age, antibiotic prophylaxis should be continued until the investigations are found to be normal. If VUR is present then prophylaxis should continue until age 5 years. Trimethoprim or nitrofurantoin are appropriate antibiotics.
- In children with no symptoms, no persistence of bacteriuria and normal renal growth on serial ultrasonography, prophylaxis can be discontinued after 5 years of age. Further UTIs should be treated early and aggressively and blood pressure and renal function monitored. Progression to CRF is unlikely in the absence of severe symptomatic infection or hypertension. It is unclear whether strategies to prevent asymptomatic bacteriuria provide long-term benefit.
- Surgical re-implantation of the ureters or endoscopic injection of Teflon may abolish VUR. It is unclear if this prevents reflux nephropathy in the longer term, but it does have a role in the management of repeated symptomatic UTIs, especially if these are causing growth retardation. It is important to remember that VUR tends to correct spontaneously as patients mature.
- In adults with established reflux nephropathy, control of hypertension and treatment of symptomatic UTIs are the mainstays of therapy. Conservative management of CRF may be needed. Female patients should be counselled carefully if pregnancy is contemplated.
- Screening of first-degree relatives by measurement of blood pressure, culture of urine and renal scanning may be appropriate.

Further reading

Eggli DF, Tulchinsky M. Scintigraphic evaluation of paediatric urinary tract infection. *Seminars in Nuclear Medicine* 1993; **23**: 199–218.
Linshaw M. Asymptomatic bacteriuria and vesicoureteral reflux in children. *Kidney International*, 1996; **50**: 312–29.
White RHR. Management of urinary tract infection and vesicoureteric reflux. *British Medical Journal*, 1990; **1**: 460–3.

Related topics of interest

Developmental abnormalities of the kidney (p. 40)
Urinary tract infection (p, 219)

RENAL ANAEMIA

Anaemia is a common feature of chronic renal failure (CRF) and contributes significantly to the morbidity of the 'uraemic syndrome'. Prolonged anaemia also contributes to the development of left ventricular hypertrophy (LVH), an important determinant of long-term prognosis. The prevalence and severity of anaemia increase as renal failure progresses. Several factors account for this anaemia, the most important being a lack of endogenous erythropoeitin. In recent years the availability of recombinant human erythropoeitin has revolutionized the treatment of renal anaemia, particularly in patients treated by dialysis.

Problems

- Poor exercise tolerance.
- Poor quality of life.
- Increased risk of LVH.
- Exposure to risks of blood transfusion.

Aetiology

1. Erythropoeitin. This is synthesized by interstitial fibroblasts in the renal cortex and directly stimulates the erythroid progenitor cells. Production declines with progressive loss of renal mass. Circulating erythropoeitin levels are then inappropriately low for the prevailing haematocrit and red cell mass declines.

2. Iron deficiency. May result from menstrual losses, poor dietary intake, low-grade gastrointestinal bleeding (not uncommon in dialysis patients), repeated blood losses during haemodialysis or frequent diagnostic tests. Iron deficiency may not manifest until after the administration of exogenous erythropoeitin increases red cell production.

3. Aluminium accumulation. This is now uncommon. It should be suspected if RBC indices are microcytic despite normal iron stores, particularly in patients who have been on haemodialysis for many years and/or have been taking aluminium-containing phosphate binders.

4. *Haematological disease.* Diseases such as myeloma or sickle-cell disease may have been the underlying cause of CRF or may coexist with it.

5. *Occult sepsis, neoplasia or other systemic disease (such as vasculitis).* These may coexist with CRF. Occult sepsis in a non-functional urinary tract is not an uncommon finding.

6. *'Uraemic' marrow depression.* This may occur as a result of severe secondary hyperparathyroidism, or because of the depressant effect on erythropoeisis of any of a number of other poorly defined 'uraemic toxins'.

Clinical assessment

- Assess likely duration and degree of CRF.
- Obtain dietary history. Enquire as to menstrual, rectal or other blood losses. Check for faecal occult blood.
- Enquire as to intake of iron and/or vitamin supplements and aluminium-containing phosphate binders.
- Establish whether sepsis, neoplasia, systemic disease or haematological disease is likely.
- Assess severity of anaemia and its impact on exercise tolerance, functional ability and quality of life.

Laboratory assessment

- Full blood count to establish haemoglobin concentration. Normochromic normocytic indices are characteristic. Hypochromic and/or microcytic indices suggest iron deficiency or aluminium accumulation.
- Iron stores should be assessed. In CRF patients, a serum ferritin of less than 100 µg/l is strongly suggestive of inadequate iron stores, which can be confirmed by marrow aspiration if necessary. Mobilizable iron stores can be assessed by measuring transferrin saturation. A value of less than 20% suggests deficiency. Serial

measurements of iron stores are particularly important following the administration of exogenous erythropoeitin.

- B_{12} and folate deficiencies are not common (especially if dialysis patients are receiving regular vitamin supplements) but should be excluded.
- Aluminium accumulation is best diagnosed by measuring the change in plasma levels that follows the infusion of desferrioxamine, which acts to mobilize tissue stores. Such tests should be done in specialized units.
- Tests to measure the level of renal function and parathyroid hormone level are appropriate. Investigations to exclude occult infection, neoplasia, systemic disease or haematological disorder may be done if clinically indicated.

Management

- General measures include limiting unnecessary venesections, encouraging an appropriate diet, avoiding aluminium-containing phosphate binders, treating water for haemodialysis by reverse osmosis to remove aluminium and identifying/correcting occult blood loss or sepsis.
- Prophylactic iron supplements should be given to all patients once they have started on dialysis. Ferrous sulphate, 200 mg daily, or a suitable alternative taken on an empty stomach, is usual. If iron deficiency exists, then a course of 200 mg three times a day or parenteral administration is necessary. Iron supplements should not be taken at the same time as phosphate binders.
- Recombinant human erythropoeitin (rHu-EPO) can be administered intravenously or subcutaneously; 40–60% of dialysis patients will require this. Increasingly, CRF patients are being treated prior to the onset of dialysis. The optimum target haemoglobin has yet to be determined. In current practice a value of 100–120 g/l is generally accepted – this may be deemed inadequate in future. A typical weekly maintenance dose of rHu-EPO would be around 100 units/kg, given in two or three divided doses.

Before commencing erythropoeitin, iron stores should be optimized and blood pressure optimally controlled.

Adverse effects include pain at the site of subcutaneous injection, flu-like symptoms, worsening of antihypertensive control (with possible risk of hypertensive seizures) and hyperkalaemia. It is uncertain whether there is also an excess risk of thrombosis in vascular access shunts.

Failure to achieve or maintain target haemoglobin usually suggests that the dose used is insufficient or that a borderline iron deficiency has been revealed by the increased needs of an enhanced erythropoeitic response. All the other factors listed above should be considered if the target is not achieved despite maximal dosage and adequate iron stores.

- Transfusion of red cell concentrate should be avoided if possible. Transfusion produces only a transient improvement in symptoms and exposes the patient to the risk of infection by blood-borne viruses, iron overload and sensitization to histocompatibility antigens (which may compromise future transplantation). In addition, blood transfusion suppresses endogenous erythropoeitin.
- Androgens were formerly given to dialysis patients and achieved a modest rise in haematocrit (possibly at the risk of hepatic damage). Their use is of historical interest only.

Current status

The principal difficulty in correcting renal anaemia now relates to the cost of providing exogenous rHu-EPO. It remains one of the more expensive products of the biotechnology industry. There is good evidence that its use significantly improves the functional ability, quality of life and cognitive function of patients with CRF or on dialysis, as well as decreasing the risk of developing LVH. Its use should now be viewed as a standard part of the integrated treatment of CRF and endstage renal disease.

Further reading

Stevens JM, Kurtz A, Echardt K-U, Winearls CG. Anaemia in chronic renal failure. In: Cameron S, Davison AM, Grünfeld J-P, Kerr D, Ritz E (eds) *Oxford Textbook of Clinical Nephrology*. Oxford: Oxford University Press, 1992; 1344–60.

Related topic of interest

Chronic renal failure (p. 31)

RENAL BIOPSY

Renal biopsy is necessary for the accurate diagnosis of parenchymal renal diseases such as glomerulonephritis and interstitial nephritis. As with any invasive procedure, it should only be performed if the risks can be justified by the benefits of accurate diagnosis.

Indications

1. Rapidly progressive glomerulonephritis. In this group of renal diseases renal function may be lost irreversibly within days. In a patient presenting with normal-sized kidneys, haematuria and proteinuria with cellular casts, and a rising serum creatinine a biopsy must be performed as soon as it is safe to do so.

2. Nephrotic syndrome. In children it is reasonable to assume that nephrotic syndrome is due to minimal change glomerulonephritis and reserve renal biopsy for patients with atypical features or poor response to steroids. In adults the differential diagnosis is much wider and treatment depends on the biopsy appearances.

3. Unexplained renal impairment. In patients with normal-sized kidneys, even if the urine sediment is unremarkable, biopsy often discloses the cause of renal impairment, although this does not always lead to a change in management.

4. Systemic disease. Renal biopsy is sometimes justified in patients to confirm a diagnosis of a systemic disease such as microscopic vasculitis, scleroderma or amyloidosis, but the yield is low unless there is haematuria, proteinuria or renal impairment.

5. Asymptomatic urinary abnormalities. Many patients are found to have haematuria, proteinuria or both on 'routine' urinalysis at medical examinations. Biopsy is usually justified in the presence of renal impairment or hypertension as these indicate that further deterioration in renal function is likely. In a normotensive patient with normal renal function the decision whether to proceed to renal biopsy often depends on what non-medical implications the result will have, for instance for employment or life insurance.

7. A.R. Failure.
8. Familial Renal Disease.

6. *Renal transplant dysfunction.* Biopsy of the transplanted kidney in the iliac fossa is easier than that of native kidneys; there is no respiratory swing and the kidney is close to the surface. Biopsy is frequently necessary to distinguish rejection from other causes of impaired function.

Contraindications

, Renal Neoplasm.
A. pyelonephritis.
, Perinephric abscess.
, obese pt.
, uraemic pt

- Coagulopathy (including abnormal template bleeding time, which should be checked in patients with significant renal impairment).
- Uncooperative patient – the patient has to stop breathing while the biopsy needle is in the kidney.
- Single kidney (unless the risks of complications, including nephrectomy, are justified).
- Reduced renal size – histology usually shows non-specific ‘endstage’ changes and it is seldom possible to alter the prognosis when the disease has advanced to the point of causing irreversible loss of renal mass.
- Severe hypertension is conventionally accepted as a contraindication.

Procedure

The patient lies prone. The lower pole of either kidney is localized, usually with ultrasound. After sterilizing the skin, local anaesthetic is introduced along the intended path of the biopsy needle as far as the capsule of the kidney (this requires a spinal needle). The biopsy needle may be advanced to the surface of the kidney in one of two ways:

- A point lying vertically over the lower pole of the kidney in inspiration is marked using ultrasound.

The needle is then advanced until it swings with respiration, indicating that the tip of the needle is on the capsule.

- The biopsy needle is advanced using 'real-time' ultrasound, allowing visualization of the needle track.

Once the needle is on the surface of the kidney, the patient is asked to stop breathing and the needle is advanced into the kidney and out again. This procedure may need to be repeated once or twice until an adequate specimen of cortex (identified by inspection using a hand-held lens) is obtained.

Complications

1. Bleeding. A small perinephric haematoma can nearly always be detected. Macroscopic haematuria may occur but is usually self-limiting. Occasionally bleeding may require blood transfusion. Very occasionally selective embolism or even nephrectomy are required to stop life-threatening bleeding.

2. Arteriovenous malformations. These are seldom clinically significant and usually close spontaneously.

3. Damage to surrounding structures. Inadvertent biopsy of neighbouring organs (liver, spleen, pancreas) may occur but should be infrequent with adequate ultrasound localization.

Further reading

Farrington K, Levison DA, Greenwood RN, Cattell WR, Baker LRI. Renal biopsy in patients with unexplained renal impairment and normal kidney size. *Quarterly Journal of Medicine*, 1989; **70**: 221–33.
Madaio M. Renal biopsy. *Kidney International*, 1990; **38**: 529–43.
Menon SK, Kirchner KA. The role of percutaneous renal biopsy in clinical nephrology. *Current Opinion in Nephrology and Hypertension*, 1993; **2**: 968–73.

Related topics of interest

RENAL INVOLVEMENT IN AMYLOIDOSIS

Amyloidosis is a systemic disease in which there is accumulation in the kidney of extracellular microfibrils which stain with Congo red. A number of biochemically distinct proteins may be identified – prognosis and treatment depend upon which protein is present and upon the pattern and severity of involvement of other organs.

Pathophysiology
- All forms of amyloid contain a glycoprotein which derives from circulating serum amyloid P (SAP). In addition, a variety of other fibril proteins are found, depending on the underlying disorder.
- Biochemical studies have identified the majority of the other deposited fibril proteins and their precursors.
- Amyloid forms β-pleated sheets which deposit as extracellular fibrils in a number of target organs. Tissue amyloid stains with Congo red and exhibits apple-green birefringence under polarized light.

Problems
- The characteristic renal presentation is with heavy proteinuria, often with nephrotic syndrome. Progressive CRF is common.
- In the earlier stages, defects of tubular function such as RTA, Fanconi syndrome or defects in urinary concentration may occur.
- Other organs may be involved.
- Cardiac involvement, with left ventricular dysfunction, tachy-dysrythmias and brady-dysrythmias, is the cause of death in up to 40% of patients with amyloidosis.
- Adrenal failure and autonomic neuropathy may cause orthostatic hypotension.
- Infiltration of the GI tract and the exocrine pancreas may cause malabsorption.
- Neuropathies without renal involvement are common in a number of inherited forms of amyloidosis.

Associated conditions	• In the past, chronic granulomatous or bacterial infections (tuberculosis, osteomyelitis and bronchiectasis) were the most common underlying disorders. These cause systemic reactive amyloidosis (formerly called 'secondary amyloidosis'). AA-amyloid is the deposited protein, derived from circulating apo-SAA protein. Treatment of biopsy specimens with permanganate causes AA-amyloid to lose its characteristic staining pattern. SAA subspecies, ranging in size from 45 to 94 amino acids, are produced by partial degradation. The different sizes may explain the variability in target organ deposition. Rheumatoid arthritis (RA), juvenile chronic rheumatoid and inflammatory bowel diseases are now the most common disorders underlying systemic reactive amyloidosis.
	• AL-amyloid deposition is associated with myeloma and other plasma cell disorders. The additional fibril proteins are immunoglobulin light chains, usually of λ type. This condition is now referred to as immunocyte-mediated amyloidosis (formerly called 'primary amyloidosis' – especially if frank myeloma was not present). Amyloid staining patterns are not affected by permanganate.
	• A number of familial forms of amyloidosis involving the kidney exist, including familial Mediterranean fever and Muckle–Wells syndrome. AA-amyloid is deposited. A range of familial amyloidotic polyneuropathy syndromes, not affecting the kidney, have been described. Mutations of the transthyretin genes produce the precursor proteins.
	• Immunocyte-mediated and RA-associated systemic reactive amyloidosis are now the most common causes of amyloidosis, which is more prevalent with increasing age.
Investigations	• A history of chronic infection or chronic inflammatory disease should be sought. Symptoms of other organ involvement may be

suggestive. Family history may be relevant, as may ethnic origin.

- Proteinuria should be quantified. Selective proteinuria (rather surprisingly) may be found. Creatinine clearance should be measured. Specific tests of tubular function may be appropriate.
- Renal size is often normal or increased on ultrasonography.
- Serum and urinary electrophoresis should be performed, with bone marrow aspiration if paraproteins are detected.
- Renal biopsy is the definitive investigation. Mesangial deposition of acidophil amorphous material without increased cellularity will be seen, usually in association with deposition in the media of blood vessels. The characteristic staining pattern will be found. Electron microscopy reveals the fibrillar nature of deposits.
- Tests of cardiac, adrenal, gastrointestinal and autonomic nervous system function may be appropriate.
- Detailed biochemical tests on the forms of amyloid proteins or precursors detected are not part of routine clinical practice.

Treatment

- Treatment is largely supportive, with the usual conservative measures for CRF. Dialysis is provided increasingly for patients with ESRF. Patients have been transplanted successfully.
- Replacement therapy for adrenal or pancreatic dysfunction may be needed. Cardiac pacing may be necessary.
- A number of uncontrolled series have shown resolution of nephrotic syndrome and amelioration of progression of CRF in patients with immunocyte-mediated amyloidosis treated by immunosuppressive regimes incorporating melphalan and prednisolone.
- Colchicine prevents attacks of familial Mediterranean fever and slows the progression of CRF in these patients.

Immunotactoid glomerulopathy

- Increasingly reports have been published of patients with renal deposition of non-amyloid fibrillar proteins. The pattern of deposition is similar to that seen in amyloidosis. Extra-renal organ involvement is unusual. A variety of terms has been coined to describe these cases, including immunotactoid glomerulopathy.
- Clinical presentation is with nephrotic syndrome, hypertension and CRF. In some series 40% of these patients progress to ESRF.

Further reading

Korbet SM, Schwartz MM, Lewis EJ. Immunotactoid glomerulopathy. *American Journal of Kidney Diseases,* 1991; **17**: 247–57.
Schwartz MM. Renal amyloidosis and other fibrillar glomerular diseases. *Current Opinion in Nephrology and Hypertension,* 1993; **2**: 238–45.

Related topics of interest

Proteinuria (p. 144)
Renal biopsy (p. 163)
Renal involvement in myeloma (p. 177)

RENAL INVOLVEMENT IN CONNECTIVE TISSUE DISEASES

Renal involvement is one of the important causes of morbidity and mortality in collagen vascular diseases and rheumatoid arthritis.

Systemic lupus erythematosus

Presenting features

It is unusual for renal disease to be the first manifestation of SLE, although some patients with membranous glomerulonephritis subsequently develop positive antinuclear factor and extra-renal disease. Renal involvement is one of the most feared complications of SLE, but detection is difficult, as the range of presenting features is broad:

- Abnormal urinalysis in a patient with SLE is due to renal involvement until proved otherwise. The probability of finding lupus nephritis is extremely high if there is evidence of complement consumption and high titre anti-dsDNA antibodies.
- Nephrotic syndrome.
- Acute renal failure – particularly in patients with active extra-renal disease.
- Chronic renal failure.

Even in patients with no clinical evidence of renal disease, renal biopsies may show all grades of lupus nephritis, but the clinical implications of this finding are uncertain.

Risk factors

The disease is more common in people of African descent; a genetic polymorphism affecting Fc receptors and causing decreased ability to remove immune complexes may be responsible.

Pathology

The WHO classification is most widely used:

1. *Class 1*. No histological abnormality.

2. *Class 2*. Mesangial glomerulonephritis with

mesangial deposition of IgG and C3, and sometimes IgM and IgA.

3. Class 3. Focal proliferative glomerulonephritis. Similar to stage 4, but not all glomeruli appear to be involved.

4. Class 4. Diffuse proliferative glomerulonephritis, with subendothelial and intramembranous deposits of IgG, C3, C1q, and usually IgA and IgM. Capillary walls may be diffusely thickened due to immune complex deposition – so-called 'wire loop' lesions. Crescents and segmental necroses may occur. A mesangiocapillary pattern may also be seen.

5. Class 5. Membranous glomerulonephritis, usually with a 'full house' of subepithelial and intramembranous immune reactants, and with variable degrees of proliferation.

6. Other features. Other features with a bearing on prognosis include tubulointerstitial inflammation and scarring and the presence of arteriolar vasculitis, both of which carry a poor prognosis.

Treatment

1. Proliferative disease. Aggressive immunosuppressive treatment is justified in patients with class 3 and 4 nephritis, who are at high risk of progressive disease. There is good evidence that cytotoxic treatment results in a better outcome than steroid treatment alone, although steroids are effective at controlling clinical flares of disease. The strongest evidence of benefit is for a regimen of intermittent monthly pulses of intravenous cyclophosphamide, initially 0.5–1.0 g/m^2, adjusted according to the leucocyte count at 10–14 days. Treatment should be continued for at least 6 months and possibly up to 2 years. Risks of cyclophosphamide treatment include haemorrhagic cystitis, reversible alopecia, premature menopause and infertility, and late malignancy. Azathioprine is useful in the maintenance of remission.

2. *Membranous disease.* There are no controlled trials in the treatment of membranous nephropathy caused by SLE (class 5 disease) but it would be reasonable to adopt a similar cytotoxic and steroid protocol to that used for idiopathic membranous nephropathy. Most clinicians would reserve treatment for patients with a progressive decline in renal function.

Drug-induced

Many drugs can cause a lupus-like syndrome, including hydralazine, procainamide and methyldopa. Renal involvement is an infrequent feature but may occur if the drug is not withdrawn when the early manifestations are present. Drug withdrawal results in resolution.

Antiphospholipid antibody syndrome

Presenting features

Antiphospholipid antibodies may occur in isolation or in association with SLE. They may be detected by screening for 'lupus anticoagulant' (*in vitro* prolongation of the APTT, not corrected with normal plasma), by detection of false positive serological tests for syphilis (VDRL), during investigation of thrombocytopenia, or by enzyme-linked immunosorbent assay for anti-cardiolipin antibodies.

These antibodies are associated with:

- Arterial and venous thromboses.
- Livedo reticularis.
- Recurrent spontaneous abortions.
- Cerebral microinfarcts.
- Glomerular thromboses and progressive renal impairment.

Management

Long-term anticoagulation is required in patients who have had clinically significant thrombosis. Aspirin may confer additional benefit, as the antibodies activate platelets. There is no evidence that immunosuppressive treatment helps.

Scleroderma

Presenting features

Renal disease is the most common cause of death in scleroderma. Proteinuria, hypertension and renal impairment are suggestive but not specific signs of renal involvement. The pathological hallmark is intimal thickening and accumulation of mucopolysaccharides in interlobular and arcuate arteries.

Scleroderma renal crisis is a syndrome of rapidly progressive oliguric renal failure and accelerated hypertension with microangiopathic haemolysis. A vicious cycle of impaired renal perfusion due to arteriolar involvement, causing renin release, acute necrotizing arteriolitis and worsening renal perfusion is responsible.

Diagnosis

Diagnosis is by clinical recognition of the skin lesions and detection of autoantibodies to extractable nuclear antigens. Renal biopsy may be necessary in cases in which the diagnosis is not obvious clinically.

Treatment

The prognosis has been transformed by the use of angiotensin-converting enzyme inhibitors, which interrupt the vicious cycle and may prevent, or even reverse, acute renal failure. Immunosuppressive treatment is ineffective.

Rheumatoid disease

Glomerulonephritis

A wide range of patterns of glomerulonephritis can occur in rheumatoid disease, including mesangial IgA disease, membranous nephropathy and (rarely) necrotizing glomerulonephritis. This is much rarer than drug-induced glomerular disease.

Drug-induced disease

1. Sodium aurothiomalate and penicillamine. These may both cause membranous nephropathy, which resolves within 2 years if the drug is withdrawn. This complication is more common in patients with the HLA-DR3 antigen. Both drugs contain thiol groups, as does captopril, which can cause similar problems. Patients receiving these drugs should be tested regularly for proteinuria. Penicillamine may also cause production of autoantibodies causing rapidly progressive glomerulonephritis and a lupus-like syndrome.

2. *Analgesics*. These may cause analgesic nephropathy when used regularly. Non-steroidal anti-inflammatory drugs may cause a variety of other renal lesions, including minimal change disease, interstitial nephritis, and precipitation of acute or chronic renal failure. Combinations of analgesics are more dangerous than single agents.

3. *Cyclosporin*. This causes dose-dependent nephrotoxicity with renal impairment and hypertension.

Amyloidosis

Long-standing rheumatoid disease may cause renal amyloidosis due to deposition of AA amyloid, which is derived from serum amyloid A protein, an acute-phase reactant. Renal amyloidosis causes proteinuria, nephrotic syndrome and then progressive renal failure. The outcome of renal replacement therapy is worse than for any other cause of renal failure, possibly due to cardiac and autonomic nervous involvement. No treatment has been shown to retard or reverse the disease.

Further reading

Black C. Scleroderma-systemic sclerosis. In: Cameron S, Davison AM, Grünfeld J-P, Kerr D, Ritz E (eds) *Oxford Textbook of Clinical Nephrology*. Oxford: Oxford University Press, 1992; 667–77.

Donadio JV, Glassock RJ. Immunosuppressive drug therapy in lupus nephritis (review). *American Journal of Kidney Diseases*, 1993; **21**: 239–50.

Piette J-C, Cacoub P, Wechsler B. Renal manifestations of the antiphospholipid syndrome. *Seminars in Arthritis and Rheumatism*, 1994; **23**: 357–66.

Related topics of interest

RENAL INVOLVEMENT IN MYELOMA

Renal disease is commonly found in patients with myeloma (up to 33% in certain autopsy series). A variety of clinical syndromes can occur, reflecting a wide variety of potential pathophysiological changes. In addition, the complications and treatment of myeloma may also lead to renal dysfunction.

Problems

- Progressive CRF with haematuria and proteinuria is the most common renal problem. Screening for myeloma is a mandatory investigation in elderly patients presenting with CRF of uncertain cause.
- Nephrotic syndrome may be the initial presentation.
- ARF may occur because of associated sepsis or hypercalcaemia. NSAIDs used to treat associated bone pain may also be implicated.
- Less commonly, tubular dysfunction presents as RTA, Fanconi syndrome or defects in urinary concentrating ability.

Pathophysiology

- Classical and specific renal lesions reflect different patterns of monoclonal light chain deposition and nephrotoxicity. The type of lesion reflects the physicochemical properties of the individual light chains. Bence-Jones proteins, first described in 1847, are identical to immunoglobulin light chain proteins.
- 'Myeloma kidney' (myeloma cast nephropathy) is the most common lesion seen. This is a non-inflammatory tubulointerstitial nephropathy occurring when light chain casts develop in the distal nephron. Tamm–Horsfall glycoprotein, a highly acidic protein synthesized in the thick ascending limb of the loop of Henle, co-aggregates with light chains. Aggregation is facilitated by lower tubular flow rates (as occurs in ECF depletion), hypercalcaemia, acidic urine and the use of radio-contrast agents. Not all light chains form casts – recent studies indicate that many of those that do are relatively resistant to degradation by locally released macrophage proteases. Intratubular obstruction leads to

progressive tubular atrophy and progressive CRF. Toxicity to the tubular cells and leakage of urine components into the interstitium also play a role.

- AL-amyloidosis occurs when light chains, or fragments of light chains, are deposited, in conjunction with amyloid P glycoprotein, as characteristic β-pleated sheets. This may affect other organs as well as the kidney. Characteristic sites of deposition are in mesangial and subepithelial regions of the glomerulus. Nodular or minimal-change glomerulopathies are seen on light microscopy. In addition, vascular deposition of AL-amyloid occurs. λ light chains are more amyloidogenic than κ light chains.

- Less commonly, non-amyloid granular deposition of light chains can cause a variety of glomerulopathies (sometimes of a proliferative nature). Heavy-chain protein deposition has also been reported.

- A wide variety of other lesions may occur. Sepsis, ECF volume depletion and hypercalcaemia may cause ATN. Hypercalcaemia may be associated with nephrocalcinosis. NSAIDs and other drugs used to treat myeloma and its complications may cause ATN or acute interstitial nephritis.

Investigations

- Immunochemical analysis, including electrophoresis, of blood and urine to identify the type of paraproteins being synthesized.
- Full blood count, skeletal survey and bone marrow examination.
- Plasma calcium.
- Dipstick urinalysis, 24 h collection of urine for creatinine clearance and protein excretion. N.B. Bence-Jones protein may not be detected by dipsticks.
- Renal biopsy, with use of appropriate stains to detect AL-amyloid, if the result is likely to influence management.
- Specific tests of tubular function, where indicated.

Management	• Specific therapy for myeloma reduces the biosynthesis of light chains and may ameliorate the renal problems in up to 20% of treated patients. However, progressive CRF is the rule, even in those who respond initially.

Management

- Specific therapy for myeloma reduces the biosynthesis of light chains and may ameliorate the renal problems in up to 20% of treated patients. However, progressive CRF is the rule, even in those who respond initially.
- Colchicine, cysteamine and vincristine reduce co-aggregation of light chains and Tamm–Horsfall proteins in experimental models – this has not been tested rigorously in patients with cast nephropathy.
- Maintenance of a high fluid intake and avoidance of radio-contrast agents and excessive use of loop diuretics.
- Urinary alkalinization, although attractive in theory, has been a disappointing intervention in clinical trials.
- Use of NSAIDs and other nephrotoxic agents should be minimized.
- Sepsis and hypercalcaemia should be treated promptly and appropriately.
- Conservative management of CRF, including the use of erythropoeitin.
- Patients with ESRF are increasingly treated by maintenance dialysis. Median survival time (from diagnosis) is reported to be about 20 months.

Further reading

Ganeval D, Rabian C, Guerin V, Pertuiset N, Landais P, Jungers P. Treatment of multiple myeloma with renal involvement. *Advances in Nephrology,* 1992; **21**: 347–70.
Sanders PW. Renal involvement in plasma cell dyscrasias. *Current Opinion in Nephrology and Hypertension,* 1993; **2**: 246–52.

Related topics of interest

Acute renal failure: general approach (p. 11)
Renal biopsy (p. 163)
Renal involvement in amyloidosis (p. 167)

RENAL OSTEODYSTROPHY

Renal osteodystrophy (ROD) is a collective term describing the mixture of pathophysiological conditions that afflict the skeletal system of patients with CRF and ESRF. ROD is most marked in patients on renal replacement therapy, but has usually begun many years previously when the GFR first starts to decline. Although not strictly a disease of bone, dialysis-associated amyloidosis (DAA) is increasingly becoming the most important symptomatic skeletal disease in dialysis patients.

Classification

- ROD is most rationally classified on the basis of a trans-iliac core bone biopsy. Prior labelling with oral tetracycline can be used to provide information on bone formation rate. In clinical practice, biopsies are performed in a minority of patients only.
- The predominant histological abnormality (in about 70% of cases) is hyperparathyroid bone disease, also called osteitis fibrosa cystica. Osteomalacia is found in about 20% and low-turnover (adynamic) bone disease in 10% of cases. A variable proportion has 'mixed' ROD with features of hyperparathyroidism and osteomalacia.

Factors controlling bone turnover

- Serum calcium levels ($[Ca^{2+}]$) are maintained primarily by the actions of activated vitamin D_3 ($1,25\text{-}(OH)_2D_3$), and parathormone (PTH).
- Vitamin D_2 (from the diet) and vitamin D_3 (from sun exposure) are activated in the liver to $25\text{-}(OH)D_3$, and in the kidney to $1,25\text{-}(OH)_2D_3$. $1,25\text{-}(OH)_2D_3$ enhances calcium uptake from the gut, promotes normal mineralization of the bone matrix and inhibits secretion of PTH, at pre-pro-PTH mRNA level.
- The enzyme responsible for final activation of $1,25\text{-}(OH)_2D_3$ is located in the mitochondria of the proximal tubule. Enzyme activity is influenced by levels of PTH, extracellular fluid $[PO_4^{2-}]$ and, possibly, acidosis.
- A matrix of stimulatory and inhibitory mechanisms links the levels of $1,25\text{-}(OH)_2D_3$, PTH, serum $[Ca^{2+}]$ and serum $[PO_4^{2-}]$. With

CRF, changes which are initially adaptive ultimately become maladaptive.

- As the morbidity associated with ROD is seen mainly in dialysis patients, the importance of preventative therapy is often overlooked by those not normally in contact with such patients.

Hyperparathyroid bone disease

- Progressive nephron loss leads to a decrease in proximal tubule 25-$(OH)D_3$ 1α-hydroxylase. This is further suppressed by raised serum $[PO_4^{2-}]$ (arising from the inability to excrete phosphate with a decreased nephron mass). Levels of 1,25-$(OH)_2D_3$ fall, leading to decreased intestinal uptake of calcium and (ultimately) towards hypocalcaemia. To counteract this, there is increased activity of the parathyroid gland. PTH levels rise when GFR has fallen to about 50 ml/min. Increased PTH enhances calcium resorption from the skeleton and is a potent phosphaturic agent. This is initially an adaptive mechanism – serum $[Ca^{2+}]$ and $[PO_4^{2-}]$ remain normal.
- When GFR is less than 30 ml/min there is a significant decrease in calcium absorption. Hypocalcaemia becomes more marked because of the decreased 1,25-$(OH)_2D_3$ levels and increased serum $[PO_4^{2-}]$. With more severe elevation of PTH, alkaline phosphatase rises, reflecting increased osteoblastic activity.
- Bone formation and destruction are both accelerated. Bone biopsy shows an increase in osteoblasts and osteoclasts, increases in the number of resorptive surfaces, an increased bone formation rate, and, occasionally, marrow fibrosis.
- Clinical features occur with advanced disease. Bone pain, myalgia and proximal myopathy occur. Pathological fractures are unusual. High levels of PTH may inhibit erythrocyte production and depress cardiac output as a direct action.
- Plain radiology shows subperiosteal resorption in the metacarpal and phalangeal bones, with

phalangeal tuft resorption and cystic lesions due to 'brown tumours'.

Treatment

- Preventative therapy involves dietary protein/phosphate restriction in the early stages of CRF. Despite normal serum $[Ca^{2+}]$ and $[PO_4^{2-}]$, PTH levels often return to normal with dietary phosphate restriction.
- As CRF advances, oral phosphate-binding agents are used. These include a variety of calcium salts and aluminium hydroxide. The use of aluminium should be minimized, however it is a more effective agent than the various calcium salts. The target $[PO_4^{2-}]$ is 1.2–1.8 mmol/l, which is not always easy to attain, especially if ROD is advanced.
- In advanced disease, metastatic calcification occurs, with joint pain and phlyctenular conjunctivitis. This is likely when the $([Ca^{2+}] \times [PO_4^{2-}])$ product is greater than 6.0 $(mmol/l)^2$. Aluminium-containing phosphate binders are unavoidable at this point. Parathyroidectomy may be required.
- Vitamin D analogues, such as calcitriol or alfacalcidol, improve calcium absorption and suppress PTH, but may cause hypercalcaemia. These should be started early in the course of CRF with a target PTH of about twice the upper limit of normal. These agents can be used to treat established hyperparathyroidism but may cause unacceptable hypercalcaemia.
- Surgical parathyroidectomy is indicated when hyperparathyroidism is refractory to these treatments. Ethanol ablation of the parathyroid nodules under ultrasound control has also been used.

Osteomalacia and aluminium-related bone disease

- The exact mechanism whereby a defect in bone mineralization occurs with CRF is unclear. Uraemic toxins may inhibit bone mineralization. Deficiency of activated vitamin D_3 contributes.
- Bone biopsy shows excessive unmineralized osteoid tissue, poor osteoclastic and osteoblastic

activity, with a decreased bone formation rate. Aluminium may be detected, laid down at the mineralization front.

- Aluminium accumulation (more of a problem in the past) from domestic water sources and aluminium-containing phosphate binders still occurs. When laid down in bone, this is probably the principal identified toxin causing the observed abnormalities.
- These are more common in diabetic, anephric and post-parathyroidectomy patients. Hypercalcaemia is a frequent problem. PTH levels may be low, possibly due to direct action on the parathyroid gland.
- Clinical features include proximal myopathy, bone pain and spontaneous fractures, especially of the ribs, spine and pelvis. Radiographical findings include fractures and demineralization.
- Prevention involves the avoidance of excessive aluminium exposure. The therapy of established disease is with desferrioxamine to chelate aluminium, avoiding the use of vitamin D analogues, using calcium-containing phosphate binders in modest quantities and possibly using lower levels of calcium in the dialysate. Severe hyperparathyroidism frequently follows successful treatment of this condition.
- It is unusual to see osteomalacia alone in ROD. Most commonly it occurs as part of a 'mixed' bone disease problem. This requires individualized therapy, depending on which form of ROD is dominant.

Adynamic bone disease

- It is unclear whether this is a specific clinical entity or even a disease. The morphological pattern seen on bone biopsy is of decreased bone turnover and decreased cellularity of bone. There is little osteoblastic and osteoclastic activity, and impaired mineralization with very small amounts of osteoid on bone surfaces is seen.
- Over-vigorous treatment of hyperparathyroidism (surgically or with vitamin D analogues) may predispose to this condition. It is also found more

frequently with moderate aluminium overload (stains for aluminium will often be positive). Some series suggest that it is more prevalent in patients treated with CAPD.

- The principal clinical problem is of hypercalcaemia, particularly if calcium-containing phosphate binders are being prescribed.
- There is no specific therapy, apart from ensuring that use of calcium salts is not excessive.

Further reading

DeBroe ME, D'Haese PC, Couttenye MM, Van Landeghern GF, Lamberts LV. New insights and strategies in the diagnosis and treatment of aluminium overload in end-stage renal failure patients. *Nephrology, Dialysis and Transplantation,* 1993; **8** (Suppl. 1): 47–50.

Delmez JA and Slatopolsky E. Hyperphosphataemia: Its consequences and treatment in patients with chronic renal disease. *American Journal of Kidney Diseases,* 1992; **19**: 303–17.

Malluche HH, Faugere MC. Renal bone disease 1990: an unmet challenge for the nephrologist. *Kidney International,* 1990; **38**: 193–211.

Related topics of interest

Chronic renal failure (p. 31)
Disorders of divalent ion metabolism (p. 49)

RENAL TRANSPLANTATION

A successful renal transplant restores a patient with renal failure to a normal life style, free from dietary restrictions and the need for regular dialysis. However, there is a price to be paid in terms of increased susceptibility to cardiovascular disease and infection. Because donor organs are limited, many patients wait for a long time before being successfully transplanted and some never receive a transplant.

Indications	• Endstage renal failure requiring dialysis. • Progressive chronic renal failure nearing endstage.
Contraindications	• Malignancy. • Active infection. • Unfit for general anaesthesia. • Extremes of age.
Living related donors	Transplanting a kidney from a sibling, parent, or (exceptionally) offspring gives better results than cadaveric donation, even if donor and recipient only share one HLA haplotype. The good results are largely due to reduction in ischaemic damage. Donors must be carefully assessed for: • Genuine altruism. • Fitness to undergo major surgery. • Absence of subclinical renal disease. • Absence of transmissible infection.
Living unrelated donors	Recently, unrelated donation from an emotionally related donor (usually a spouse) has been shown to be successful, even in the absence of close HLA matching. In Western countries, pre-operative work-up of potential unrelated donors requires exacting checks to ensure that the offer to donate is truly altruistic and is tightly regulated by law. In some developing countries, transplantation from paid unrelated donors is the dominant form of renal replacement therapy.
Cadaveric donation	This is the source of most transplanted kidneys in the UK and USA but is rare in Japan and in Muslim and Hindu countries. The vast majority of organs are

retrieved from 'beating heart donors' in which there is evidence of irreversible brainstem damage ('brainstem death'), diagnosis of which requires:

- Coma due to structural damage of known cause.
- Absence of drugs or conditions (e.g. hypothermia) which could impair brainstem function or reflexes.
- Absent respiratory drive despite hypoxia and hypercarbia.
- Absent brainstem reflexes, including corneal reflex, doll's eye reflex, vestibulo–ocular reflex, gag and cough reflexes.

Absence of transmissible infection or malignancy are required and the kidneys should be capable of working normally.

Kidneys are normally retrieved after *in situ* perfusion with an ice-cold electrolyte solution while the donor's heart is still beating and then kept on ice until implantation.

Transplant immunology

1. Blood group. The donor kidney has to be ABO compatible, and preferably identical. Matching for other blood group antigens is unnecessary.

2. HLA typing. Identification of the HLA type of an individual currently relies on the use of serum samples from donors known to have antibodies against certain antigens. Some sera are cross-reactive against families of similar 'broad antigens'. Molecular techniques may soon allow more accurate typing.

3. HLA matching. The risk of graft failure is directly related to the number of antigens it carries which are foreign to the recipient. Computerized matching schemes operate in most countries to allow the 'best' recipient to be found for a particular kidney, although these procedures increase the cold ischaemic time. Some recipients may be offered poorly matched grafts to avoid continuing problems with dialysis.

4. *Cytotoxic antibody screening.* Serum samples from the patient are tested for their ability to kill lymphocytes (in the presence of complement) from a panel of donors. Pre-formed IgG antibodies to a defined HLA antigen are highly predictive of acute rejection of an organ carrying that antigen, and may be the result of previous pregnancy, blood transfusion, or an earlier transplant. Autoantibodies may cause false positive results.

5. *Cross-matching.* Stored and fresh sera from the potential recipient are incubated with lymphocytes from the donor. Complement-dependent lysis predicts 'hyperacute rejection' and means that the transplant should not go ahead. A positive cross-match with B cells (which carry HLA class II antigens and a higher density of class I antigens) with a negative T-cell cross-match is of less certain predictive value. Fluorescent-activated cell sorter (FACS) cross-matching is a more sensitive way of identifying anti-HLA antigens.

Immunosuppression

1. *Cyclosporin.* This is the mainstay of most regimens. It acts by preventing T-cell recruitment in response to new antigens. Its major disadvantage is nephrotoxicity. Acute nephrotoxicity causes a fall in GFR and hypertension and is caused by renal vasoconstriction; in the longer term this may cause irreversible ischaemic damage. Absorption from the gut is variable, and numerous drugs interfere with cyclosporin metabolism. Monitoring of blood levels is useful, but there is no clear separation between therapeutic and toxic levels.

2. *Steroids.* These are used in most regimens although some centres achieve good results without long-term steroid use. High-dose methyl-prednisolone remains the most widely used treatment to reverse acute rejection.

3. *Azathioprine.* This drug acts on the bone marrow to reduce lymphocyte proliferation and has

a less specific immunosuppressive effect than cyclosporin. Allergic reactions and hepatitis occur rarely. Its action is potentiated by allopurinol, addition of which may precipitate bone marrow aplasia. It is often used as 'triple therapy' with steroids and cyclosporin, particularly in high-risk patients.

4. *Biological agents.* These include polyclonal anti-thymocyte globulin and a range of monoclonal antibodies against antigens involved in signalling between lymphocytes and in antigen recognition and binding. These are powerful agents and may be used as initial prophylactic treatment in patients at high risk of acute rejection and for reversal of steroid-resistant acute rejection. In the future it is hoped that biological agents will be developed which will induce donor-specific tolerance.

5. *New agents.* These include tacrolimus and sirolimus, which have similar actions to cyslosporin but may be more potent; deoxyspergualin; and mycophenylate, which acts in a similar way to azathioprine.

Complications

1. *Acute rejection.* This is common, and may occur even in well-matched grafts. Other causes of acute loss of graft function include acute tubular necrosis, cyclosporin nephrotoxicity, obstruction and ascending infection. Evidence of renal swelling and increased resistance to arterial blood flow are suggestive but not diagnostic. Renal biopsy is required to confirm the diagnosis, although aspiration cytology is used in some centres. Rejection usually responds to high-dose methylprednisolone; steroid-resistant rejection is usually treated with a biological agent and may prompt intensification of background immunosuppressive treatment.

2. *Chronic renal allograft dysfunction.* This is also termed chronic rejection, and is characterized by

progressive loss of renal function, proteinuria and hypertension. Renal biopsy may show glomerular, arteriolar and interstitial changes and is required to exclude recurrent disease or cyclosporin nephrotoxicity. It appears to be caused by a combination of humoral immunity and repair processes following early nephron damage, but is unaffected by intensified immunosuppression.

3. *Technical problems.* These may lead to arterial or venous thrombosis or to ureteric necrosis.

4. *Opportunistic infections.* These include cytomegalovirus (CMV) infection, other viral infections and *Pneumocystis* pneumonia. Prophylaxis against CMV should be used if either donor or recipient has evidence of past infection.

5. *Recurrence of primary disease.* This may occur in glomerulonephritis (particularly mesangiocapillary GN and primary focal segmental glomerulosclerosis) but does not always result in loss of renal function. Rapidly progressive glomerulonephritis may recur, particularly in anti-glomerular basement membrane disease. Primary hyperoxaluria should be treated with combined hepatic and kidney transplantation to avoid recurrence.

6. *Malignancy.* There is an increased risk of lymphoproliferative disease, particularly after intensive immunosuppression; many of these diseases are initiated by uncontrolled lymphocyte proliferation in response to Epstein–Barr virus infection. There is also a greatly increased risk of skin malignancies and of cervical cancer.

7. *Cardiovascular disease.* Both hypertension and hyperlipidaemia are very common after transplantation, particularly with cyclosporin treatment, and many recipients of a successful graft die prematurely from cardiovascular disease.

Calcium-channel antagonists have the advantage that they may also ameliorate cyclosporin nephrotoxicity. Lipid-lowering drugs should be used with caution because of an increased risk of muscle toxicity when used with cyclosporin.

Outcome

Outcome depends on HLA matching, co-morbid conditions, and pre-existing HLA-specific antibodies. One-year graft survival should be:

* 80–90% for first cadaveric grafts.
* >90% for living related grafts.
* 75% for highly sensitized patients and those with co-morbid conditions such as diabetes.

Despite major advances in prevention of acute rejection, 10-year survival is only approximately 50%, depending on initial function and HLA matching.

Further reading

Suthanthiran M, Strom TB. Renal transplantation. *New England Journal of Medicine*, 1994; **331**: 365–76.

Related topics of interest

Drug induced renal disease (p. 57)
Focal segmental glomerulosclerosis (p. 77)
Other inherited causes of renal disease (p. 129)
Post-infectious and mesangiocapillary glomerulonephritis (p. 139)
Urolithiasis (p. 229)

RENAL TUBULAR ACIDOSIS

A renal tubular acidosis (RTA) the urine is found to be inappropriately alkaline in the presence of a systemic acidaemia. A heterogeneous group of disorders with a common feature of tubular dysfunction may manifest as RTA.

Diagnosis

- Should be suspected with a hyperchloraemic, metabolic acidosis with normal anion gap. There should be no evidence of GI fluid loss, no intravenous infusion of cationic amino acids (such as arginine and lysine) and no acute changes in respiratory function.
- Classically, renal function is normal. However, specific syndromes can be recognized in the setting of mildly impaired renal function.
- Associated electrolyte abnormalities are common and may be the more important pathophysiological derangement.
- Urinary acidification tests are rarely performed for clinical purposes.
- Primary and familial cases of RTA are reported. Acquired RTA occurs in a wide range of conditions.

Classification

- Many systems of classification have been proposed. There are essentially three broad categories. These can be distinguished fairly easily on clinical grounds. The underlying cellular abnormalities are often complex and diverse.

- Hypokalaemic Proximal RTA (formerly type II)
- Hypokalaemic Distal RTA (formerly type I)
- Hyperkalaemic Distal RTA (formerly type IV)

- Mixed disorders also exist.

Tests of urinary acidification

- If a freshly voided morning urine sample has a pH below 5.3 then there is no problem with distal acidification mechanisms.
- If urine pH is above 5.3 in the presence of acidaemia, renal tubular acidosis is present. If the diagnosis is suspected in a patient whose baseline venous bicarbonate is normal, acidaemia is

induced by oral ingestion of ammonium chloride (0.1 mmol/kg) and urine pH measured over the subsequent 6–8 h. If distal mechanisms are intact, urine pH should fall below 5.3.

- A more elaborate test involves measurement of urinary pCO_2 after bicarbonate loading to raise urine pH to or above 7.5. With normal acidification mechanisms, urinary pCO_2 exceeds blood pCO_2 by at least 30 mmHg. This set is unreliable in the presence of metabolic alkalosis.

- The urinary anion gap ($Na^+ + K^+ - Cl^-$) is a rough measure of urinary ammonium (NH_4^+) secretion. This gap is usually negative. A positive value suggests that distal ammonium secretion is impaired.

- Following a single dose of a loop diuretic, urinary pH falls by about 1 unit (in response to increased delivery of sodium to the distal nephron) if distal acidification mechanisms are normal.

- Proximal tubular acidification is measured by assessing the fractional excretion of bicarbonate when plasma bicarbonate is normal. This should not exceed 5%.

Hypokalaemic proximal RTA

- The characteristic defect is excessive fractional excretion of bicarbonate (>15%) in the presence of normal or low plasma bicarbonate concentration. Distal mechanisms to excrete H+ remain intact. Severe acidaemia is therefore uncommon, as urinary pH can fall below 5.3 in the face of more marked acidaemia. Plasma bicarbonate levels of 14–18 mmol/l are characteristic.

- Aminoaciduria, glycosuria and phosphaturia are common. Hypophosphataemia and vitamin D-resistant rickets may coexist.

- Urinary citrate excretion is normal and nephrocalcinosis is uncommon. Osteomalacia is a frequently associated finding.

- The associated hypokalaemia is usually mild, but may fall with the administration of alkali.

- The amount of alkali needed to achieve normalization of plasma bicarbonate is high, with patients requiring up to 10-15 mmol/kg/day. Alkali administration may improve growth during childhood. It should be given with potassium supplements.
- This commonly presents in childhood. Cystinosis, tyrosinaemia and hereditary fructose intolerance are all associated with proximal RTA. Wilson's disease, heavy metal poisoning, amyloidosis, multiple myeloma, medullary cystic disease and administration of outdate tetracycline have all been reported to cause proximal RTA. It is also seen in the early stages after renal transplantation and in nephrotic syndrome.
- The long-term prognosis for renal function is good.

Hypokalaemic distal RTA

- The characteristic defect is an inability to decrease urinary pH below 5.3 even in the presence of severe acidaemia. Plasma bicarbonate levels of less than 10 mmol/l are therefore characteristic.
- Aminoaciduria, glycosuria and phosphaturia are uncommon.
- Clinical problems include muscle and skeletal symptoms, weakness and even paralysis, due to the associated severe hypokalaemia.
- Nephrocalcinosis is a characteristic feature. Fifty per cent of patients suffer recurrent urolithiasis with calcium phosphate stones. This reflects mobilization of skeletal calcium in the face of severe acidaemia, with marked hypercalciuria. Decreased urinary citrate excretion adds to the risk of stone formation. Osteomalacia is uncommon.
- Alkali requirements are of the order of 1–2 mmol/kg/day. Potassium citrate may be an appropriate choice. With these doses symptoms, hypokalaemia and urolithiasis may improve. Alkali therapy should be targeted to reduce hypercalciuria, as this is the principal threat to longer term renal function.

- Hypercalcaemia, myeloma, amyloidosis, SLE, Sjögren's syndrome and medullary sponge kidney are reported to cause hypokalaemic distal RTA. There is an association with hepatic cirrhosis. Lithium and amphotericin therapy may be implicated and it is seen with renal transplant rejection.
- The long-term prognosis for renal function is more guarded than for proximal RTA because of nephrocalcinosis.

Hyperkalaemic distal RTA

- The characteristic defect is an inability to decrease urinary pH below 5.3. As the level of acidaemia is usually mild, it may be necessary to perform acid-loading tests to reveal this feature. Plasma bicarbonate levels of 15–20 mmol/l are characteristic.
- Aminoaciduria, glycosuria and phosphaturia are uncommon.
- This frequently occurs with a mild degree of renal impairment. Hyperkalaemia (inappropriate for the level of renal impairment) rather than acidaemia is the usual clinical problem.
- Nephrocalcinosis, hypercalciuria, decreased urinary citrate excretion and osteomalacia are uncommon. Systemic hypertension and oedema are often present.
- Various cellular abnormalities underlie this condition.
- There may be a primary defect in ammoniagenesis, but hyperkalaemia itself is a cause of decreased ammoniagenesis.
- In some cases chronic ECF volume expansion leads to suppression of the renin-angiotensin-aldosterone (RAA) axis – so-called hypo-reninaemic hypoaldosteronism. This may be part of the spectrum of normal ageing, but is frequently seen with diabetes mellitus and chronic interstitial nephritis.
- Treatment may need to incorporate dietary potassium restriction, alkali therapy, diuretic therapy or mineralocorticoid administration, depending on the associated abnormalities.

- This type of RTA occurs in obstructive uropathy, analgesic nephropathy, sickle-cell disease, amyloidosis, myeloma, lead nephropathy, SLE and diabetic nephropathy. It is associated with adrenal insufficiency and AIDS. Potassium-sparing diuretics, NSAIDs, ACEIs and cyclosporin all cause hyperkalaemic distal RTA. Prolonged heparin therapy, with inhibition of adrenal 11-b–hydroxylase, may also be implicated.
- The long-term prognosis for renal function reflects the prognosis of the associated disease.

Further reading

Garella S. Clinical acid/base disorders. In: Cameron JS, Davison AM, Grünfeld J-P, Kerr D, Ritz E (eds) Oxford Textbook of Clinical Nephrology. Oxford: Oxford University Press, 1992; 917–65.

Nairns RG, Jones ER, Townsend R, Goodkin DA, Shay RJ. Metabolic acid-base disorders: pathophysiology, classification and treatment. In: Arieff AI and DeFronzo RA (eds) *Fluid, Electrolyte and Acid-Base Disorders*. New York: Churchill Livingstone, 1985; 269–384.

Related topics of interest

RENAL VASCULAR DISEASE

Ischaemic renal damage is difficult to recognize clinically, yet it is an important cause of renal failure, particularly in the elderly.

Renal artery stenosis

Haemodynamically significant stenosis of the renal artery has two major effects: renovascular hypertension as a result of increased renin release from the ischaemic kidney, and progressive renal failure as a result of ischaemic atrophy. Because hypertension of any cause results in structural changes in resistance vessels, long-standing renovascular hypertension may not be corrected by successful renal revascularization. Once ischaemic atrophy has occurred, this too is irreversible. However, as with coronary artery disease, the decision on when to proceed to invasive investigation with a view to renal revascularization remains controversial, because investigation and treatment also carry risks.

Causes

1. Fibromuscular dysplasia. Medial thickening and intimal fibrosis alternating with segments of aneurysmal dilatation cause the 'beaded' appearance which is usually diagnostic on angiography. The disease occurs in early adult life and affects females more often than males. Other vascular beds, such as the mesenteric arteries, may also be involved. The pathogenesis is unknown.

2. Atherosclerosis. Involvement of the renal artery is usually a late stage of systemic atherosclerosis. Up to 30% of patients undergoing coronary or lower limb angiography have evidence of some renal artery involvement. Renal artery stenosis may be ostial (at the origin from the aorta); affecting the main renal artery; or may involve intra-renal branches. The renal artery may also be 'pinched off' at its origin by involvement in the wall of an aortic aneurysm.

Presentation

1. Hypertension. Renovascular disease should be suspected in hypertensive patients with:

- Early or late onset.
- No family history of essential hypertension.
- Accelerated phase hypertension.

- Hypertension resistant to conventional therapy.
- Acute decline in renal function associated with ACE inhibitor use.
- Hyponatraemia and evidence of volume depletion (due to unilateral disease causing pressure-natriuresis in the unaffected kidney).
- Otherwise unexplained renal impairment.

Because hypertension may cause progression of atherosclerosis, it is often impossible to distinguish cause from effect in an individual with vascular disease and hypertension, unless the blood pressure is known only to have risen recently.

2. *Renal impairment.* Renovascular disease should be considered in patients with renal impairment, even in the absence of hypertension, if there is evidence of vascular disease elsewhere and no evidence of another cause of renal failure. Ischaemic renal disease is one of the few causes of renal impairment with negative urinalysis, although it can cause significant proteinuria.

3. *Recurrent pulmonary oedema with normal left ventricular function.* This is a feature of bilateral renal artery stenosis and is attributable to sodium and water retention: decreased renal perfusion pressure results in decreased natriuresis, resulting in worsening hypertension, which directly impairs left ventricular emptying. Left ventricular hypertrophy, causing diastolic dysfunction, may also contribute.

Investigation

The diagnosis may be suggested by asymmetry of renal size on ultrasound or IVU, or of renal excretion on IVU, but neither investigation is sensitive or specific, particularly for bilateral renal artery stenosis.

1. *Captopril-enhanced renography.* This is widely used as a screening test. Prolongation of isotope transit time on one side compared to the other suggests functionally important stenosis and predicts the response to renal revascularization. The test is

not reliable in the presence of renal impairment, because this usually means that there is bilateral disease, which does not result in asymmetry of isotope clearance.

2. Duplex scanning. Detection of high-velocity blood flow distal to a stenosis is highly suggestive of renal artery stenosis. The technique is highly time-consuming and observer-dependent, and reliable results have only been reported from a few centres.

3. Renal vein renin. Comparison of renin production from the two kidneys should, in theory, indicate which kidney is causing hypertension in renovascular disease. In practice, measurement of renal vein renin concentration (which does not necessarily parallel production rate because of variability in renal vein flow rate) has been unreliable in predicting the blood pressure response to revascularization in most studies.

4. Angiography. Detailed images of the renal arteries may be obtained by conventional intra-arterial contrast injection (with digital subtraction to reduce the amount of contrast required) or by magnetic resonance angiography. The latter may overestimate stenoses and is only validated in a few centres. Angiography is clearly the 'gold standard' for the identification of stenoses.

Indications for treatment

Revascularization should nearly always be considered in fibromuscular disease. In atherosclerotic disease revascularization should be considered in patients whose blood pressure cannot be satisfactorily controlled with drugs or whose renal function is deteriorating rapidly. It is more difficult to decide whether to proceed to investigation in patients with well-controlled hypertension and stable renal impairment. The risks of progressive renal ischaemic damage in this situation are finely balanced against the risks of invasive investigation and treatment.

Treatment

1. Blood pressure. This should be controlled without ACE inhibitors or angiotensin II antagonists.

2. Conservative. Neither lipid–lowering treatment nor aspirin has (yet) been shown to delay progression of renal artery stenosis, but use of both drugs is often jusitified by the presence of atherosclerotic vascular disease elsewhere.

3. Angioplasty. This is the treatment of choice in fibromuscular dysplasia. Long-term follow-up is required to detect restenosis or contralateral disease. In atherosclerotic disease the results (both in reducing blood pressure and restoring renal function) are less predictable. Insertion of metallic stents seems likely to prove a useful adjunct to angioplasty, particularly in ostial lesions.

4. Surgery. Several operations are available, including endarterectomy, vein grafting, and anastomosis of the diseased renal artery to the hepatic or splenic artery. The choice very much depends on local expertise. Surgery for renal artery disease should only be performed in specialist centres.

Thromboembolism

Embolic infarction of the kidneys is rare but probably under-recognized. The risk factors are the same as those for embolism elsewhere – atrial fibrillation, dilated cardiomyopathy, valvular disease, and severe aortic atherosclerosis. Emboli to the kidneys may also come from thrombus within an abdominal aortic aneurysm.

Clinical features

- Flank pain – may be mistaken for renal colic.
- Fever, acute-phase response.
- Macroscopic haematuria.
- Acute renal failure (particularly if bilateral or to a single functioning kidney).
- Raised LDH.

Course and treatment	Most episodes resolve leaving a cortical scar, but massive embolism can result in dialysis-dependent renal failure. Depending on the source of emboli, long-term anticoagulation may be required.

Atheromatous embolism

Atheromatous ('cholesterol') embolism is a complication of severe atherosclerosis which may mimic systemic vasculitis and is under-recognized. It is caused by embolism of fragments of ulcerated atherosclerotic plaque.

Clinical features	• Fever. • Acute-phase response – raised ESR, viscosity. • Hypocomplentaemia. • Eosinophilia. • Livedo reticularis. • Acute renal impairment.
Causes	• Spontaneous. • Following intra-arterial catheterization, for example coronary angiography. • Following streptokinase or anticoagulation (? by preventing fibrin deposition on an ulcerated plaque).
Diagnosis	Biopsy of affected skin or of the kidney shows occluded arterioles, with pathognomonic needle-shaped clefts where cholesterol crystals have dissolved out during processing.
Treatment	Dialysis may be required if renal damage is severe. Anticoagulants and angiography should be avoided. Recovery of renal function, with recanalization of occluded arterioles, has been reported.

Further reading

Jacobson HR, Breyer JA. Ischaemic renal disease. In: Cameron S, Davison AM, Grünfeld J-P, Kerr D, Ritz E (eds) *Oxford Textbook of Clinical Nephrology*. Oxford: Oxford University Press, 1992; 1077–84.

Mann J, Allenberg J-R, Reisch C, Dietz R, Weber M, Luft FC. Renovascular hypertension. In: Cameron S, Davison AM, Grünfeld J-P, Kerr D, Ritz E (eds)

Oxford Textbook of Clinical Nephrology. Oxford: Oxford University Press, 1992; 2096–117.

Tomson CRV. *Hypertensive Nephropathy.* London: Science Press, 1996.

Related topics of interest

THE KIDNEY AND HYPERTENSION

The kidney has a crucial role in blood pressure regulation both via control of renin release and via control of circulating volume. Normally, a rise in blood pressure results in a rise in sodium and water excretion, returning blood pressure to normal (the 'pressure-natriuresis relationship'). For hypertension to be sustained, this pressure-natriuresis relationship has to be re-set. This is true whether the hypertension is 'essential' or secondary to primary renal disease, endocrine disease, or sympathetic overactivity. However, for practical purposes, it is important to determine whether hypertension is 'primary' or 'secondary', because many of the secondary causes require different or additional treatment.

Hypertension secondary to renal disease

Pathogenesis

1. Renin/angiotensin system. Decreased perfusion of the juxtaglomerular apparatus causes renin release, resulting in increased formation of angiotensin II, a potent vasoconstrictor.

2 Circulating volume. Even minor degrees of renal disease may cause sodium and water retention and result in expansion of the circulating volume, causing hypertension without necessarily causing other signs of volume overload such as oedema and raised venous pressure.

3. Increased sympathetic nerve traffic. This has been demonstrated recently in hypertensive patients with renal failure, and renal sympathetic stimulation is known to cause sodium retention.

4. Other factors. Decreased intrarenal production of nitric oxide reduces sodium excretion as blood pressure rises. Decreased production of medullipin, a potent vasodilator lipid produced in the renal medulla, may also contribute to hypertension. The importance of these factors is uncertain.

Causes and investigation

1. Glomerulonephritis. Any type of glomerulonephritis, including minimal change disease, can cause hypertension, which will remit if the disease can be treated. A renal biopsy should be considered if urinalysis is abnormal

2. *Diabetic nephropathy.* Hypertension is an early feature of diabetic renal disease. In a patient with a long history of diabetes and retinopathy it is often safe to assume, without biopsy, that proteinuria and hypertension are due to diabetic nephropathy.

3. *Polycystic kidney disease.* Hypertension may be the presenting feature in this disease. A family history is not always obtained. The diagnosis is best confirmed by ultrasound.

4. *Reflux nephropathy.* A history of urinary infection is not always obtained. Urinalysis may give normal results. Intravenous urography is the investigation of choice.

5. *Renal artery stenosis.* Fibromuscular renal artery dysplasia should be suspected particularly in young females, and atherosclerotic renal vascular disease in patients with coronary or peripheral vascular disease. Captopril-enhanced isotope renography is a useful screening tool in patients with normal renal function: the gold standard remains angiography.

6. *Obstructive uropathy.* High-pressure chronic retention of urine is a reversible cause of hypertension in men. A tense, painless bladder should be sought even in the absence of typical symptoms. Ultrasound shows hydronephrosis and hydroureter.

7. *Scleroderma.* Renal involvement in this disease may be unsuspected until the development of a 'scleroderma renal crisis' with accelerated hypertension and renal failure. Urinalysis may be normal but often shows proteinuria, and haematuria if accelerated hypertension has developed. Renal biopsy is diagnostic, although the appearances can

be difficult to distinguish from those seen in primary accelerated hypertension.

8. Page kidney. This involves compression of the kidney by perinephric haematoma or subsequent fibrosis following trauma, causing high renin hypertension.

Who to investigate?

A full history and examination with urinalysis for glucose, protein and blood should be obtained in all patients with hypertension and will identify many patients whose hypertension is possibly of renal origin. Even if these give no clues, further investigation for the diseases listed above should be considered if a hypertensive patient has:

- Accelerated hypertension.
- No family history of hypertension.
- Presentation at less than 30 or more than 60 years of age.
- Impaired renal function.
- Atherosclerosis.

Treatment

The underlying condition should be corrected where possible. If cure is not possible, hypertension should be controlled with drugs. Hypertension secondary to renal disease is associated with an increased risk of progressive renal failure, and effective treatment reduces this risk.

1. Loop diuretics. Effective in volume-dependent hypertension: high doses may be necessary in renal impairment. Thiazide diuretics are ineffective anti-hypertensives in patients with renal disease.

2. Calcium-channel blockers. Often effective.

3. Angiotensin-converting enzyme inhibitors. Normalize intraglomerular pressure and reduce proteinuria, and may be more effective in reducing the risk of progressive renal failure than equipotent doses of other antihypertensives in proteinuric patients. They are contraindicated in renal artery stenosis, where they may produce an irreversible decline in renal function.

4. β-blockers. These are frequently used, but may require dosage adjustment.

Renal disease in essential hypertension

'Benign' essential nephrosclerosis

Essential hypertension, by definition, is not associated with renal impairment or proteinuria at presentation. However, renal impairment and/or proteinuria may occasionally develop as a late result of essential hypertension, particularly if blood pressure control is poor. The evidence is confusing, largely because definitive proof would require prolonged follow-up of a large group of hypertensive patients in whom underlying primary renal disease had been excluded by exhaustive investigation.

1. Epidemiology. Long-term follow-up of patients screened for the MRFIT study shows that the risk of developing renal failure is directly related to initial blood pressure (and also to smoking habits and blood cholesterol).

2. Risk factors. 'Hypertensive nephrosclerosis' is more commonly cited as a cause of endstage renal failure in Afro-Americans than in Caucasian Americans. Although this could be due to poorer blood pressure control, small-scale treatment studies suggest an increased susceptibility even if blood pressure is well controlled.

3. Clinical presentation. Slowly progressive renal dysfunction in a patient with long-standing hypertension suggests hypertensive nephrosclerosis. Microalbuminuria is common in hypertension and does not necessarily predict progressive renal disease. Heavy, even nephrotic-range, proteinuria may occur. It is important to exclude potentially treatable causes, including renal artery stenosis.

4. Pathology. Renal biopsy shows thickening, tortuosity and hyalinosis of arterioles; tubular atrophy and intersitial fibrosis; and glomerulosclerosis without evidence of glomerulonephritis or immune reactants.

Accelerated hypertension Any type of hypertension may, if untreated, lead to an accelerated phase. A secondary cause is found in up to 50% of patients; glomerulonephritis is an important cause in patients under 35 and atherosclerotic renal vascular disease in patients over 60.

1. Presentation. Severe hypertension, headache, visual loss, abdominal pain, and renal failure occur. Urinalysis shows haematuria and proteinuria and fundoscopy shows haemorrhages and exudates, with or without papilloedema.

2. Pathology. Renal biopsy shows fibrinoid necrosis of arterioles.

3. Pathogenesis. A vicious cycle of arteriolar damage, leading to decreased renal perfusion, increased renin release and further worsening of hypertension is the cause.

4. Outcome. Untreated, accelerated hypertension has a high mortality (largely from stroke) and causes irreversible renal impairment; spontaneous resolution is rare but can occur.

5. Treatment. Blood pressure should be lowered gradually: overenthusiastic antihypertensive treatment can precipitate ischaemic stroke. Parenteral treatment is seldom justified.

Further reading

Tomson CRV. Hypertensive Nephropathy. London: Science Press, 1996.

Wilkinson R. Clinical approach to hypertension. In: Cameron JS, Davison AM, Grünfeld J-P, Kerr DNS, Ritz E (eds) *Oxford Textbook of Clinical Nephrology*. Oxford: Oxford University Press, 1992; 2047–58.

Related topics of interest

Autosomal dominant polycystic kidney disease (p. 26)
Chronic renal failure (p. 31)
Diabetic nephropathy (p. 44)
Glomerulonephritis: general approach (p. 81)
Renal vascular disease (p. 196)

THE KIDNEY IN PREGNANCY

Major changes in renal function occur during normal pregnancy. Pre-existing hypertension or chronic renal disease may prevent these adaptive changes and result in life-threatening pre-eclampsia. Hypertension occurs in 10% of pregnancies, most of which are otherwise uncomplicated. However, 1 in 2000 pregnancies is complicated by eclampsia, which is the most common cause of maternal death. In patients with pre-existing chronic renal disease, pregnancy may result in worsening renal function and progression to endstage renal failure.

Normal physiology

Normal pregnancy results in:

- Increased cardiac output.
- Decreased peripheral resistance.
- Fall in blood pressure during first trimester, with a rise to pre-pregnancy levels towards term.
- Increased plasma volume.
- Increases in renal plasma flow and glomerular filtration rate (up to 180 ml/min).
- Increased fractional urate clearance, returning towards normal at term.

Hypertension in pregnancy

Definition

Blood pressure falls in normal pregnancy. A rise in blood pressure of greater than 15 mmHg diastolic or 30 mmHg diastolic from measurement in early pregnancy is taken as significant, as is a blood pressure (confirmed on subsequent measurements) of greater than 140/90 mmHg.

Measurement

Although identification of the fourth Korotkoff sound is difficult and poorly reproducible, this is how diastolic blood pressure has been defined in most of the studies of hypertension in pregnancy. Lower action limits will need to be defined if the fifth sound is adopted.

Chronic hypertension

This is defined as:

- known history of hypertension before conception; or

- blood pressure greater than 140/90 mmHg before 20 weeks of pregnancy; or
- failure of hypertension to resolve within 6 weeks of delivery.

Most cases are due to essential hypertension, but it is important to exclude treatable causes of secondary hypertension: undetected phaeochromocytoma causes a maternal mortality of 50% and the prognosis for the fetus is poor in Cushing's syndrome.

Transient hypertension

A rise in blood pressure in the third trimester without proteinuria or other features of pre-eclampsia is relatively benign, but may recur in subsequent pregnancies and predict the later development of sustained essential hypertension. It can only be differentiated from pre-eclampsia in retrospect.

Pre-eclampsia

This syndrome usually, but not always, causes hypertension. By definition, hypertension develops after 20 weeks' gestation and usually after 35 weeks. It is nearly always associated with proteinuria (>0.3 g/day), which may reach nephrotic proportions. By definition, pre-eclampsia may progress to full-blown eclampsia (convulsions), but the rate of progression may be so fast that hypertension and proteinuria remain undected until the onset of convulsions. Over 40% of cases of eclampsia occur post-partum.

1. Pathogenesis. Failure of trophoblastic invasion, leading to placental hypoperfusion, is thought to cause activation of the coagulation cascade and the placental renin-angiotensin system. The exact pathogenesis of the widespread organ dysfunction remains uncertain but endothelial dysfunction caused by substances released from the hypoxic placenta would explain many of the features.

2. Risk factors.

- First pregnancy.
- Subsequent pregnancy by a new father ('primipaternity').

- Short period of sexual co-habitation prior to conception.
- Family history of pre-eclampsia (particularly if the patient's mother was pre-eclamptic in the gestation of the patient).
- Asthma.
- Chronic hypertension.
- Pre-existing disease.

3. Symptoms. The early stages are asymptomatic. Rapidly worsening oedema, headache, visual disturbances, right upper quadrant abdominal pain and apprehensiveness all suggest an impending crisis.

4. Signs. Hyperreflexia, abdominal tenderness and retinal arteriolar spasm may occur.

5. Investigation. There is no 100% reliable diagnostic test. Decreased urinary kallikrein excretion may be of predictive value. Rising serum urate, falling platelet count and increasing 24 h urinary protein excretion are suggestive. Renal biopsy shows glomerular endotheliosis, a lesion unique to pre-eclampsia, but is not routinely used unless it is important to exclude underlying primary renal disease.

6. Crises. Pre-eclampsia is a multisystem disease:

- Convulsions (= eclampsia).
- Cerebral haemorrhage (particularly in patients with chronic hypertension).
- HELLP syndrome: haemolysis, elevated liver enzymes, low platelets.
- Disseminated intravascular coagulation.
- Acute renal failure (acute tubular or cortical necrosis, haemolytic uraemic syndrome).
- Hepatic rupture.
- Cerebral haemorrhage.
- Fetal asphyxia and intra-uterine death.

7. Prevention. Antihypertensive treatment in patients with chronic hypertension reduces the risk of pre-eclampsia if this is defined by a rise in blood pressure, but has not been shown to reduce the risk of proteinuria or of the crises listed above. Aspirin has been widely used but the largest study to date (the CLASP study) did not confirm a preventive effect.

8. *Management.* This consist of:

- Delivery as soon as possible.
- Parenteral magnesium sulphate, which has recently been shown to be superior to phenytoin in preventing convulsions in pre-eclampsia and in preventing further convulsions in eclampsia, probably by reversing cerebral vasospasm.

Treatment

1. Chronic hypertension. Hypertension in the second trimester is associated with an increased risk of stillbirth, intra-uterine growth retardation and pre-eclampsia. However, it is not known for certain whether treatment of hypertension during pregnancy reduces these risks, as hypertension may result from impaired placental perfusion, rather than being its cause; antihypertensive treatment, particularly if it lowers cardiac output, might further impair fetal perfusion. In addition, some antihypertensive drugs may be teratogenic. Hypertension may be complicated by accelerated hypertension, hypertensive heart failure and stroke in the mother. The balance of evidence favours treating hypertension, mostly because this will reduce the risk of severe hypertension in the mother. The antihypertensives thought to be safest are:

- methyldopa,
- clonidine,
- labetalol.

The use of diuretics and calcium-channel blockers is controversial. ACE inhibitors cause birth defects and are contraindicated.

2. Transient hypertension and pre-eclamptic hypertension. The aim of treatment is to prevent hypertensive encephalopathy and cerebral haemorrhage; it is uncertain whether antihypertensive treatment reduces the risk of an eclamptic crisis. Methyldopa and labetalol are widely used; calcium-channel blockers are also effective. Diuretics should be avoided because plasma volume is often contracted; volume expanders have even been used to correct hypertension, but require careful monitoring. Parenteral hydralazine or labetalol are used for severe hypertension or rapidly rising blood pressure.

Pregnancy in patients with primary renal disease

Effects on pregnancy

Pre-existing renal disease, even in the absence of hypertension, increases the risk of pre-eclampsia. Renal impairment at conception is associated with intra-uterine growth retardation and death. Patients with recurrent pre-eclampsia should undergo investigation for underlying renal diseases, including reflux nephropathy and chronic glomerulonephritis.

Effects on renal function

The risk of progressive decline in renal function as a result of pregnancy is low in patients with normal renal function at conception, although proteinuria may increase markedly. In patients with renal impairment, whatever the cause, there is a significant risk of acclerated deterioration in renal function, particularly if proteinuria is also present. Pregnancy should be avoided, or consideration given to termination, if serum creatinine is above 200 mmol/l at conception. Successful pregnancies in patients on dialysis have been reported but are exceptional.

Specific diseases

1. Systemic lupus erythematosus. Lupus nephritis may present for the first time during pregnancy, and patients with previous disease may experience severe flares of disease, sometimes with acute renal failure. These complications are unpredictable.

Patients with known lupus nephritis should be advised against pregnancy unless the disease is quiescent, and even then should continue immunosuppressive treatment during pregnancy.

2. *Antiphospholipid antibody syndrome.* This is associated with recurrent abortions, which may be preventable with aspirin, and with an increased risk of renal impairment caused by thrombotic microangiopathy.

3. *Scleroderma.* Pregnancy may precipitate a scleroderma renal crisis, particularly as ACE inhibitors cannot be used during pregnancy.

4. *Renal transplantation.* The risk of acute decline in renal function depend on pre-pregnancy renal function, and are similar to those in patients with disease of their native kidneys. The risk of developmental abnormalities in patients taking azathioprine and cyclosporin is relatively low.

Acute renal failure in pregnancy

Incidence

Acute renal failure complicating pregnancy has become very rare (less than 1 in 10 000 pregnancies), mostly because of the decline in the number of septic abortions.

Causes

- Septic abortion causing DIC and acute tubular necrosis.
- Acute pyelonephritis - common in pregnancy and more commonly leads to a reduction in GFR than in non-pregnant patients.
- Hypovolaemia such as uterine bleeding, hyperemesis gravidarum.
- Pre-eclampsia and eclamptic crises, including the HELLP syndrome.
- Complicating liver failure in acute fatty liver of pregnancy.
- Idiopathic post-partum haemolytic uraemic syndrome.
- Disorders unrelated to pregnancy, including rapidly progressive glomerulonephritis.

Clinical course   In most cases, renal failure is due to acute tubular necrosis, and is fully reversible. However, acute hypovolaemia during late pregnancy is the most common cause of acute bilateral cortical necrosis, which usually results in irreversible renal failure.

Further reading

Collins R, Wallenburg HCS. Pharmacological prevention and treatment of hypertensive disorders in pregnancy. In: Chalmers I, Enkin M, Keirse MJNC (eds) *Effective Care in Pregnancy and Childbirth*, Volume 1. Oxford: Oxford University Press, 1989; 512–33.

Lindheimer MD, Davison JM (eds) Renal disease in pregnancy. *Ballières Clinical Obstetrics and Gynaecology*, 1994; **8** (2), London: Ballières Tinall, 1994.

Redman CWG, Roberts JM. Management of pre-eclampsia. Lancet, 1993: **341**: 1451–4.

Roberts JM, Redman CWG. Pre-eclampsia: more than pregnancy-induced hypertension. *Lancet*, 1993; **341**: 1447–51.

Related topics of interest

Acute renal failure: general approach (p. 11)
Glomerulonephritis: general approach (p. 81)
Reflux nephropathy (p. 154)
Renal involvement in connective tissue diseases (p. 171)
Urinary tract infection (p. 219)

URINALYSIS AND URINE MICROSCOPY

Careful examination of the urine can give valuable information on renal function and on the presence of renal inflammation. Dipstick urinalysis only costs a few pence and should be considered as much part of the routine clinical examination as measurement of the blood pressure.

Appearance

Colour

Urine is usually a yellowish colour. The depth of the colour is only a very rough guide to urine concentration; numerous pigments contribute to the colour of urine and their intake is very variable. Red urine is usually due to haematuria, but can follow intake of beetroot ('beeturia') in iron deficiency. Urine may change colour on standing in patients with porphyria and on L-dopa.

Clarity

Urine is usually crystal clear. Cloudy urine may be due to urine infection with pyuria, crystalluria (usually phosphate crystals in alkaline urine) or (rarely) chyluria.

Dipstick testing

Many different dipsticks are available and it is therefore important to know which one has been used. 'Urine NAD' is meaningless without this information. Tests for ketones, bilirubin, and urobilinogen do not give information about renal function or disease and will not be discussed further here.

Blood

This test relies on the presence of haemoglobin. Discrete, punctate colour change indicates the presence of red cells, whereas diffuse colour change may indicate free haemoglobin, but the distinction is unreliable in practice. Myoglobin cross-reacts in the assay; a strongly positive dipstick test for blood in muddy brown urine with no red cells visible on microscopy strongly suggests myoglobinuria. False positive tests may also be caused by contamination of urine by iodine or hypochlorite but this is rare. Bacterial peroxidase may also cause positive tests, but the test is not a reliable method of detecting urinary infection. The most common cause of a positive dipstick test with negative urine microscopy is lysis of red cells while awaiting microscopy.

Protein

This test utilizes a pH-sensitive indicator, buffered within the strip, whose colour-change point is altered by protein binding. The test is sensitive to albumin, but other urinary proteins (e.g. light chains) do not produce a colour change. A protein concentration of around 300 mg/l is required for a colour change to be detected. Normal urine contains a small amount of protein, so highly concentrated urine may cause a 1+ reaction. Bacterial urine infection may produce a positive test. Strongly positive tests nearly always indicate renal disease. False positive tests may occur if urine pH is less than 7.0.

pH

These dipsticks rely on pH-sensitive dyes. Knowledge of urine pH is rarely helpful. Alkaline urine occurs in urine infection with urease-producing organisms such as *Proteus* spp., which cause infection stones. A urine pH >5.3 in the presence of systemic acidosis is diagnostic of renal tubular acidosis.

Nitrite

This test is usually positive in urine infection, but not all organisms produce nitrite.

Leucocyte esterase

This test detects pyuria, which is usually (but not always) present in significant urine infection.

'Microalbuminuria'

Dipsticks are now available which detect much lower concentrations of albumin than can be detected by conventional dipsticks. These employ specific enzymatic assays for albumin, and are useful in the detection of so-called 'microalbuminuria' – elevated albumin excretion in the range 30–300 mg/24 h. These tests are expensive and, at present, operator-dependent.

Urine microscopy

Microscopy of urine has been termed 'the liquid biopsy'. Detection of pus cells aids in the interpretation of urine cultures and is usually performed by junior scientific staff in the microbiology laboratory using bright-field illumination. More detailed information can be obtained from careful examination of fresh urine under phase-contrast illumination and requires experienced staff. Occasionally, staining of the urine sediment may be required.

Pyuria

Pus cells are usually, but not invariably, present in infected urine. Sterile pyuria can be due to chlamydial lower urinary tract infection, to partially treated bacterial urine infection, or to papillary necrosis, stones or renal tuberculosis.

Eosinophiluria

Eosinophils may be found in the urine in acute interstitial nephritis. Accurate identification requires staining.

Epithelial cells

These cells are larger than leucocytes and are shed in increased numbers in acute tubular necrosis.

Red cells

These are usually easily recognized as biconcave disks. However, glomerular bleeding results in shrinkage and deformity of the cells as they pass through the loop of Henle. Recognition of these deformed red cells is strongly suggestive of glomerular bleeding, although their absence does not preclude glomerulonephritis. If large numbers of red cells are present, examination of urine in a Coulter counter allows automated analysis of the size distribution of red cells: if the mean cell volume is significantly less than that of a concurrent blood sample, a glomerular origin is likely. These distinctions are less reliable in dilute or alkaline urine.

Casts

These are formed by precipitation of Tamm–Horsfall glycoprotein, a component of normal urine, within the tubular lumen.

1. Hyaline casts. These are found in normal urine and contain Tamm–Horsfall glycoprotein only. Increased numbers are seen after diuresis.

2. Granular casts. These are casts of cell debris and are abnormal but do not indicate the exact site of the abnormality.

3. White cell casts. Diagnostic of acute pyelonephritis.

4. Red cell casts. Diagnostic of the presence of red cells within the tubules, and usually indicate glomerular haematuria.

5. Broad or waxy casts. These are formed in dilated atrophic tubules and indicate chronic renal disease.

Further reading

Fogazzi GB, Passerini P, Ponticelli C, Ritz E. *The Urinary Sediment. An Integrated View*. London: Chapman & Hall Medical, 1994.

Related topics of interest

Acute renal failure: general approach (p. 11)
Glomerulonephritis: general approach (p. 81)
Haematuria (p. 84)
Interstitial nephritis (p. 113)
Renal tubular acidosis (p. 191)

URINARY TRACT INFECTION

Urinary tract infection (UTI) is a common cause of morbidity, which frequently follows a recurrent course. In certain circumstances, urinary infection can contribute to progressive deterioration in renal function.

Clinical symptom complexes
- Acute cystitis presents with frequency, dysuria and suprapubic pain, often associated with fever and systemic malaise.
- Acute pyelonephritis presents with fever, loin pain and systemic upset, with or without associated lower tract symptoms.
- Frequency-dysuria ('urethral') syndrome occurs in young and middle-aged women. Systemic features are unusual.
- Non-specific symptoms of irritability and fever in children.
- Asymptomatic bacteriuria.

Classification
- Distinguish between complicated and uncomplicated UTIs. Complicated UTIs are those occurring in an anatomically abnormal urinary tract, in patients with urinary tract stones, in catheterized patients and in immunosuppressed patients.
- Distinguish between community-acquired and nosocomial infections. Most community-acquired UTIs are due to *E. coli*. Nosocomial infections may be due to a variety of organisms and are often associated with complicated UTIs.

Aetiology
- The majority of organisms causing UTI originate in the patient's own bowel. Invasion is predominantly via the urethra, but may be haematogenous in infants.
- Mechanical and contact factors may be important, especially with the urethral syndrome. These include sexual intercourse, nylon underwear, spermicides, atrophic vaginitis, rubber sensitivity and scratching. Inappropriate and repeated antibiotic therapy may increase rather than decrease the incidence of UTI.

- Bacterial virulence factors are important. Only a few groups of *E. coli* serotypes are virulent to the urinary tract. *Escherichia coli* expressing MS (mannose-sensitive) and MR (mannose-resistant) fimbriae can bind to urothelial cells, possibly protecting them from elimination during micturition. Lipid A lipopolysaccharide (endotoxin) inhibits ureteric peristalsis. Biotin production protects against high urinary osmolality.
- Host factors are important. Glycosuria allows more rapid bacterial growth. Vesico-ureteric reflux, urinary tract stones and incomplete bladder emptying facilitate infection. Non-secretor blood group status is associated with an increased risk of infection. The shorter female urethra is more easily ascended. Pregnancy-associated changes in the urinary tract render it especially vulnerable to ascending infection.
- Evidence is accumulating that many patients, especially those with lower tract symptoms, may have relatively low urinary bacterial counts (as few as 20 000 cfu/ml) with associated infection of the urethra or peri-urethral glands. Alternatively infection may be with fastidious organisms, such as *Chlamydia*.

Epidemiology

- One per cent of boys and 3% of girls suffer a symptomatic UTI before their teens. Incidence of symptomatic UTI is much higher in females, except at the extremes of age.
- Recurrent UTIs are more prevalent in females. In males, even a single UTI suggests an underlying structural abnormality or chronic prostatitis.
- Asymptomatic bacteriuria is found in 1–2% of schoolgirls and 5% of sexually active young women. It occurs in 3.5% of normal pregnancies, and in 30% of elderly patients of both sexes.

Organisms

- *Escherichia coli* is the most common organism, occurring in up to 75% of cases. In boys *Proteus* species may cause up to 40% of cases. Coagulase-negative staphylococci are frequently found in sexually active young women with lower tract symptoms.

- In complicated UTI, organisms such as *Proteus*, *Klebsiella* and *Pseudomonas* may be implicated.

Investigations

- Proper collection of urine samples is important. The midstream urine technique is appropriate for adults and older children but may not be much better than the simpler clean-catch technique. Suprapubic aspiration or adhering a sterile plastic bag to the perineum is appropriate in infants.
- The initial sample obtained on urethral catheterization may be informative, but it is difficult to interpret findings on samples obtained from a catheter which has been *in situ* for some time.
- To speed diagnosis, a plastic dipslide with blood agar on one side and cystine lactose-deficient (CLED) medium on the other may be dipped into freshly collected urine and transported to the laboratory.
- Quantitative culture of urine has been the gold standard for diagnosis of UTI since 1956, when Kass introduced the concept of 'significant bacteriuria'. Bacterial counts of greater than 100 000 colony-forming units/ml were formerly felt to reflect infection rather than colonization or contamination. It is now clear that much lower counts (20 000 cfu/ml) can be associated with symptomatic UTI, especially in women. Pure growth of a single organism with associated pyuria confirms that infection is present.
- Antibiotic sensitivities are determined by applying antibiotic-impregnated discs to culture media after plating of urine samples.
- Microscopy of fresh uncentrifuged urine is used to detect leucocytes (pyuria). Gram stain may help to identify organisms before culture results are available.
- Screening tests using dipstick tests for nitrates or catalase activity are available. A positive test for nitrates has a specificity of greater than 90% but a sensitivity of about 50%, compared with a 92%

sensitivity and 95% specificity for Gram staining and urine microscopy.

- Radiological investigations to exclude structural abnormalities or urolithiasis may be appropriate, and are mandatory in infants because of the potential existence of vesico-ureteric reflux or other problems. Ultrasonography and intravenous urography may be selected, as may voiding cystourethrography.
- DMSA scans may illustrate transient defects at the site of renal infection which may persist for several weeks.

Management

- General measures include advice on good perineal hygiene, regular and complete micturition habit, good fluid intake and avoidance of irritants.
- Patients who are systemically unwell will require supportive care which will include i.v. rehydration and analgesia.
- The agent, route of administration and duration of antibacterial therapy will depend upon the clinical circumstances and the results of microbiological culture.
- For uncomplicated lower tract infection, single doses or 3–5-day courses of oral therapy have been advocated. Shorter courses seem to be as effective with fewer side-effects but with a slightly higher relapse rate. Trimethoprim, cephalexin or amoxycillin are appropriate choices.
- For complicated or upper tract infections with marked systemic symptoms, initial parenteral therapy with subsequent oral therapy for 5–14 days may be necessary. Extended spectrum cephalosporins, co-amoxiclav or quinolones may be appropriate.
- Infection in an obstructed urinary tract may require percutaneous or surgical drainage.
- Recurrent infections may be minimized by long-term prophylaxis with a single daily dose of trimethoprim or nitrofurantoin. The safety of very long-term use of nitrofurantoin is unclear.

- Instrumentation of the urinary tract should always be covered with antibiotic therapy. Urinary catheterization should be used only for appropriate indications and long-term placement avoided if possible.
- There is little evidence that treatment of asymptomatic bacteriuria in the elderly is beneficial. However, bacteriuria should always be treated in pregnancy as it will be followed by symptomatic infection in at least 30% of cases.

Complications
- UTI may be followed by bacteraemia and severe systemic inflammatory response syndrome (SIRS). Localized problems such as pyonephrosis or renal carbuncle may occur.
- Although urinary sepsis alone is unlikely to lead to chronic renal damage, its occurrence in the setting of structural abnormalities (especially vesico-ureteric reflux) may contribute to the development of renal insufficiency in the longer term.

Further reading

Stamm WE. Criteria for the diagnosis of urinary tract infection and for the assessment of therapeutic effectiveness. *Infection,* 1992; **20**, (Suppl. 3): S151–S154.
Stamm WE, Hooton TM. Management of urinary tract infections in adults. *New England Journal of Medicine,* 1993; **329**: 1328–34.

Related topics of interest

URINARY TRACT MASSES AND CYSTS

Renal masses and cysts may be detected as incidental findings during abdominal ultrasound examinations or may be found during investigation of haematuria.

Renal parenchymal masses

Wilms' tumour

This is an embryonic tumour ('nephroblastoma'). Its frequency is increased in several developmental abnormalities; mutations in two separate genes on chromosome 11 (WT1, WT2) have been identified, but mutations on other chromosomes may also be associated. More than 90% present before the age of 7, usually as the incidental finding of an abdominal mass. Bilateral tumours may occur. Surgical resection may need to be followed by chemotherapy and/or radiotherapy, depending on staging.

Neuroblastoma

This is also a childhood tumour, of sympathetic nervous system origin, which may be intrarenal.

Renal cell carcinoma

This tumour, also called hypernephroma, is the most common renal tumour of adults, and is derived from proximal tubular cells. Tumours may be multiple and occasionally bilateral. The tumour is more common in smokers and in von Hippel–Lindau syndrome, in which there is deletion of a tumour suppressor gene on chromosome 3p. Sporadic renal cell carcinoma may also involve genetic mutations on other chromosomes.

1. Presenting symptoms and signs. These include painless macroscopic haematuria, flank pain (rare, and late), palpable mass, hypertension, malaise, fever, weight loss and symptomatic anaemia.

2. Laboratory findings. These include raised ESR and plasma viscosity, abnormal liver enzymes, hypercalcaemia, normochromic anaemia and occasionally erythrocytosis. All of these may occur without overt metastases and resolve after nephrectomy.

3. Diagnosis. This is usually made by ultrasound. CT scanning is helpful in confirming the diagnosis and for assessing local spread and lymph node involvement. Chest radiography and isotope bone scan are required for staging.

4. Treatment. Radical surgical excision, unless both kidneys or a single functioning kidney are involved, in which case partial nephrectomy may be considered. Radiotherapy and chemotherapy are relatively ineffective. Metastatic disease may be treated with α-interferon, interleukin-2 and 5-fluorouracil but the response rate is poor and side-effects frequent. Older patients may derive symptomatic benefit from medroxyprogesterone acetate.

Oncocytomas

These are rare tumours of tubular cells with densely packed mitochondria. CT scanning may show a central hypodense stellate 'scar'. Treatment is by surgical removal.

Simple renal cysts

Occasional renal cysts are common incidental findings in older patients undergoing renal imaging. Multiple cysts should raise the possibility of adult polycystic kidney disease, even if there is no family history, and may also occur in von Hippel–Lindau disease and tuberous sclerosis. Cyst aspiration cytology and CT scanning may be necessary to differentiate benign from malignant cysts.

Acquired cystic disease

Multiple cysts may develop in kidneys which have sustained irreversible damage from chronic renal disease, such as glomerulonephritis and hypertensive nephrosclerosis. Usually they are only detected after years of dialysis, but may occur in patients with chronic renal failure who are not yet at endstage. Apart from duration of chronic renal failure, risk factors include male sex and black race. Renal anaemia may improve, due to increased erythropoietin production. Multiple renal tumours develop in up to 40% of patients, more commonly in men, and may cause macroscopic haematuria, but death from metastatic disease is rare.

Hamartomas

Multiple renal angiomyolipomata, containing fat and smooth muscle and blood vessels, may occur in isolation or with tuberous sclerosis. The high fat content is diagnostic on CT scanning. Lesions over 4 cm may rupture, causing massive retroperitoneal bleeding; selective angiographic embolization should be considered.

Infective masses

1. Xanthogranulomatous pyelonephritis. This is a rare form of acute pyelonephritis caused by the combination of ascending infection and ureteric obstruction. Large numbers of lipid-laden macrophages accumulate. Extension to perinephric tissue, systemic symptoms, radiological appearances and even the histological features may mimic renal adenocarcinoma. Treatment is by nephrectomy.

2. Malakoplakia. This is a rare granulomatous condition caused by infection, usually in the urinary tract, combined with an acquired defect in phagocytosis. Histological appearances are characteristic. Prolonged treatment with ciprofloxacin is the treatment of choice.

Tumours of the pelvis, ureter and lower urinary tract

Transitional cell carcinoma

These may occur in the renal pelvis and ureter or in the bladder.

1. Presenting features. Most present with painless macroscopic haematuria. Screening for microscopic haematuria in elderly men may allow earlier detection. Invasive bladder tumours often present with advanced disease, including obstructive renal failure.

2. Risk factors. These include cigarette smoking, analgesic abuse, exposure to petrochemicals, prolonged treatment with cyclophosphamide, Balkan nephropathy and 'Chinese herb nephropathy'.

3. Diagnosis. Upper urinary tract tumours are diagnosed by imaging, usually intravenous urography and/or retrograde pyelography. Cytological examination of urine or brushings taken at ureteric catheterization may be helpful. Lower urinary tract tumours are best investigated by cystoscopy and biopsy.

4. Treatment. Treatment of upper tract tumours is surgical resection. Low-grade (non-invasive) bladder tumours may regress after intravesical BCG, mitomycin, or other cytotoxics but require life-long surveillance with check cystoscopies. High-grade bladder tumours are treated with radical cystectomy, where this is a feasible option, or by radiotherapy.

Squamous cell carcinoma

These are much rarer than transitional cell tumours and usually arise in areas of chronic inflammation caused by stones (e.g. staghorn calculi) or indwelling urinary catheters; there is a high incidence in paraplegic patients with neurogenic bladder. Treatment is surgical.

Prostatic carcinoma

Prostate cancer is the second most common malignancy to cause death in men and is the most frequently diagnosed male cancer. It may present with bladder outflow symptoms or with bilateral obstructive uropathy (due to spread within the bladder wall, involving the ureteric orifices), but is often asymptomatic in its early stages and presents late with metastatic bone disease. Asymptomatic disease is common in elderly men, who should be observed without treatment if they have a life expectancy less than 10 years. Symptomatic disease, and asymptomatic disease in younger men, may be treated with radical prostatectomy (if the disease is localized), radiotherapy or hormonal treatment (surgical castration or anti-androgen treatment). The benefits of early detection by screening (by digital examination and measurement of prostate-specific antigen) are uncertain.

Further reading

Catalona WJ. Management of cancer of the prostate. *New England Journal of Medicine*, 1994; **331**: 996–1004.

Dawson C, Whitfield H. Urological malignancy – II: Urothelial tumours. *British Medical Journal*, 1996; **312**: 1090–4.

Dawson C, Whitfield H. Urological malignancy – III: Renal and testicular carcinoma. *British Medical Journal*, 1996; **312**: 1146– 8.

Related topics of interest

Analgesic nephropathy (p. 21)
Autosomal dominant polycystic kidney disease (p. 26)
Imaging of the urinary tract (p. 110)
Interstitial nephritis (p. 113)
Other inherited causes of renal disease (p. 129)

UROLITHIASIS

Formation of calculi within the urinary tract and their subsequent passage is a very common clinical problem, causing substantial morbidity, consuming considerable health care resources and occasionally leading to chronic renal damage.

Epidemiology

- Urinary tract stones are found in 1–3% of autopsies. The lifetime risk of urolithiasis is 5–10% for women and almost 20% for men. Peak incidence of a first stone event is in the fifth decade. Stones are more common in Caucasian patients and in those from higher socio-economic strata.
- Higher consumption of animal protein is associated with a higher prevalence of renal stones.
- Ten per cent of stone events lead to hospital admission. About 5% of stones require surgical treatment. Fifty per cent of patients suffer a first recurrence within 5 years. Seventy-five per cent have had a recurrence within 20 years.

Stone formation

- Stones consist of crystal systems within a complex matrix skeleton.
- A mixture of calcium oxalate and calcium phosphate is the most common (40%) type of stone. Pure calcium oxalate (25%) and calcium phosphate (7%) stones are also found. 'Struvite' (magnesium ammonium phosphate and calcium phosphate) accounts for 20% of stones. Uric acid (7%), cystine (1%) and xanthine (<1%) stones are uncommon.
- Stone formation is influenced by the level of saturation of the urine, the presence of inhibitors and the possibility of spontaneous organic nucleation. Urine must be supersaturated to allow crystal nucleation. However, many non-stone-formers also have supersaturated urine.
- Specific inhibitors prevent crystal nucleation in supersaturated urine. Citrate is an important inhibitor, particularly of calcium phosphate stone formation. Hypocitraturia is more common in

stone formers. Magnesium also inhibits calcium phosphate stone formation. Calcium oxalate stone formation is inhibited by nephrocalcin and Tamm–Horsfall protein.

- Heterogeneous nucleation may occur on to a conglomeration of organic material. The composition of this material is unclear. Tamm–Horsfall protein may be a component.

Presentation

- Caliceal stones present with recurrent dull flank pain.
- Stones in the renal pelvis present with bouts of severe pain as the stone impacts on the pelvi-ureteric junction (PUJ).
- Ureteric stones present with severe colicky pain and haematuria.
- Haematuria may be macroscopic or microscopic.
- Stones or 'gravel' may be passed spontaneously.
- Relapsing urinary tract infection or severe sepsis may occur.
- Stones obstructing a single ureter may cause ARF or pyonephrosis.
- Staghorn calculi may lead to chronic renal failure.

Investigations

- Plain KUB radiography has a sensitivity of *c.* 75% for stones. Conventional tomography increases this to 85%.
- Ultrasonography has a similar sensitivity for stones larger than 2.5 mm. Smaller stones can be missed. Non-opaque stones are best detected by ultrasonography, but intravenous urography (IVU) may be necessary for ureteric stones.
- Size and number of stones can be evaluated by IVU, which will also provide information on associated drainage problems.
- Chemical analysis, including polarization microscopy, of any stone passed is most important.
- Careful evaluation identifies an abnormality in the risk factor profile for stone formation in the majority of patients.

- Quantitative dietary history and history of drug ingestion (particularly OTC preparations containing vitamin C, vitamin D and calcium) should be taken.
- Dipstick urinalysis, urine culture, plasma calcium, phosphate, urate and creatinine estimation are necessary. Daily urinary excretion of calcium, urate, oxalate and citrate should be assessed by 24 h collection. This should be done as an outpatient on a usual (not hospital) diet.
- PTH should be measured in hypercalcaemic patients. If this is normal and the patient remains hypercalcaemic, plasma angiotensin converting enzyme levels can be measured, a raised level suggests sarcoidosis.

Idiopathic calcium urolithiasis

- This term describes a complex of abnormalities found in the majority of stone formers. These include a variable combination of increased urinary excretion of calcium, oxalate, uric acid and sodium with a decreased urinary excretion of citrate, magnesium, nephrocalcin and Tamm–Horsfall protein.
- Hypercalciuria (>0.1 mmol/kg/day) is frequent (30–50%), but not a universal feature. Some patients show raised vitamin D concentrations and/or increased intestinal calcium absorption. A minority show accelerated bone turnover, negative calcium balance and reduced bone density. Familial hypercalciuria is well recognized.
- Urinary oxalate is derived mainly from endogenous synthesis. Testosterone increases production by increasing hepatic glycolic acid oxidase activity. Males are five times more likely to develop calcium oxalate stones. Up to 40% of urinary oxalate is derived from dietary ascorbic acid. Leafy vegetables, beetroots, and animal proteins are rich sources. Normally only 5% of dietary oxalate is absorbed. This increases to 10% if dietary calcium is restricted.

- Urinary citrate excretion is very sensitive to changes in urinary and cellular pH. Hypocitraturia is found in systemic acidoses and with potassium and magnesium depletion.

Other underlying disorders
- Hyperparathyroidism is found in 95% of patients with hypercalcaemia, hypercalciuria and renal stones. However, stones occur in only 10% of all patients with hyperparathyroidism. Parathyroidectomy effectively abolishes the risk of stone formation in 95% of patients.
- Struvite stones occur with chronic infection by urease-producing micro-organisms. Ureolysis produces ammonia, bicarbonate and carbonate. Many organisms produce urease. The most frequently (75%) isolated organisms are *Proteus* species. *Escherichia coli* rarely produces urease. Culture of stone material may be necessary to identify the organism involved. Struvite stones often form staghorn calculi. They occur in 5–10% of patients with spinal cord injury and in 5–30% of patients with ileal conduits. Antibiotic therapy is rarely of benefit in preventing stone formation. There is evidence that surgical clearance of these stones may help to preserve renal function and prevent further urolithiasis.
- Renal stones develop in 7–10% of patients with inflammatory bowel disease. ECF depletion with decreased urine volume leads to increased supersaturation for all types of crystals. Urinary inhibitors such as citrate, magnesium, phosphate and sulphate are low.
- Calcium oxalate stones develop in 10–20% of patients with small bowel disease or ileal bypass. Malabsorption of fat leads to the formation of calcium–fat complexes in the intestine. Calcium oxalate complexes thus decrease and oxalate absorption increases, leading to hyperoxaluria. Malabsorption of bile damages the colonic epithelium, further increasing oxalate absorption.
- Uric acid stones develop in patients with other bicarbonate-losing gastrointestinal diseases.

Acidic urine of low volume with hypocitraturia is found.

- Triamterene and sulphonamides can crystallize in the urinary tract.
- Hypokalaemic distal RTA is commonly associated with calcium phosphate stone formation.
- Fifty per cent of patients with xanthinuria (xanthine oxidase deficiency) present with radiolucent xanthine stones. Serum uric acid is low and urinary uric acid excretion is negligible.
- Other inherited conditions, such as cystinuria and primary hyperoxaluria, also present with renal stones.

Follow-up

- The objective is to render patients clinically and metabolically inactive. Clinical activity is defined as a new symptomatic episode. Metabolic activity is defined as the appearance or increase in size of stones on plain KUB radiography and/or the passage of gravel.
- Having established the underlying risk factors, general measures are instituted, with specific measures when appropriate.

Medical treatment

- High fluid intake is the single most important intervention, especially in hot climates. Patients with urine outputs over 2000 ml/day tend to be metabolically inactive and have fewer recurrent stone events. Fluid intake should be spaced throughout the 24 h period to prevent urine concentration overnight.
- High dietary intake of animal proteins and oxalate-containing foods should be avoided. There is no evidence that restriction of calcium intake is of value, as any benefit is offset by an increase in absorption of oxalate. Decreasing oxalate intake may be of greater value. Decreasing sodium intake may be of value, especially in patients with hypercalciuria.
- Thiazide diuretics decrease urinary calcium excretion and may decrease urinary oxalate excretion. Studies suggest a decreased recurrence

rate in both hypercalciuric and normocalciuric patients. This may not be effective in primary hyperabsorptive hypercalciuria or in those with high dietary sodium intake.

- Potassium citrate (often in combination with magnesium citrate) may be useful in hypocitraturic patients and in hypokalaemic distal RTA.
- Allopurinol may decrease recurrence rates. It is unclear if this applies other than in hyperuricosuric patients.
- Several treatments have been used with little evidence of benefit. Sodium cellulose phosphate may decrease gastrointestinal absorption of calcium, but may also increase oxalate absorption and decrease magnesium absorption. Potassium acid phosphate, pyridoxine and orthophosphate have also been used.

ESWL

- ESWL (extra-corporeal shock wave lithotripsy) is now the treatment of choice in 60–90% of patents with renal or ureteric stones. Percutaneous nephrolithotomy and ureteroscopic manipulation may be needed for more complicated stones. ESWL is best used for symptomatic or obstructive stones. Stones larger than 3 cm may require percutaneous lithotripsy in addition. With smaller stones, 90% of patients should be stone-free at 3 months

Further reading

Coe FL, Parks JH, Asplin JR. The pathogenesis and treatment of kidney stones. *New England Journal of Medicine*, 1992; **327**: 1141–52.
Preminger GM. Renal calculi: pathogenesis, diagnosis and medical treatment. *Seminars in Nephrology*, 1992; **12**: 200–16.
Tomson CRV. Prevention of recurrent calcium stones: a rational approach. *British Journal of Urology*, 1995; **76**: 419–24.

Related topics of interest

Disorders of divalent ion metabolism (p. 49)   Renal tubular acidosis (p. 191)
Urinary tract infection (p. 219)

VIRAL DISEASES AND THE KIDNEY

A number of viral infections can cause renal disease, either by direct invasion of the renal parenchyma or indirectly by immune complex-mediated damage. Most are relatively uncommon. Viral illnesses are also important causes of illness in immunocompromised patients with renal disease or renal transplants.

Hepatitis B virus (HBV)

- HBV is a global public health problem, with more than 300 million chronic carriers. Prevalence of carriage varies from 0.1 to 15% in different geographical regions. Infection during infancy or childhood is more likely to lead to carrier status.
- A clear association with glomerular disease has been established. Glomerular capillary deposition of different viral components has been identified. Membranous glomerulopathy is the classical morphological pattern. A mesangio-capillary pattern also occurs. There may be an increased incidence of IgA nephropathy in chronic HBV carriers.
- HBV-associated GN is much less frequent than many of the other complications of chronic HBV carriage, such as cirrhosis or hepatocellular carcinoma. It is more likely to be found in children and is uncommon in areas with a low prevalence of carriage.
- Clinical presentation is usually with nephrotic syndrome.
- The natural history is not completely understood. In many cases the nephrotic syndrome resolves spontaneously. Some cases progress to CRF. Treatment with steroids is felt to be unwise because of the potential to facilitate active viral replication in the liver. α-interferon therapy has been administered with disappointing results. Large well-designed trials of treatment regimens have not been conducted.

Hepatitis C virus (HCV)

- HCV infection is usually transmitted by blood transfusion or i.v. drug abuse. It is the most common cause of non-A, non-B hepatitis in dialysis patients. It may also present primarily with renal disease.

- HCV infection is associated with mixed essential cryoglobulinaemia and with a non-cryoglobulinaemic mesangiocapillary glomerulonephritis (often without evidence of liver disease).

Cytomegalovirus (CMV)

- The most usual manifestation of CMV infection in renal disease is as an illness presenting early after renal transplantation. This may be especially severe if the recipient is seronegative, has received an organ from a seropositive donor and receives biological agent immunosuppression.
- CMV is implicated as a facilitator of increased rates of allograft rejection. It may also cause an interstitial nephritis in transplant recipients. Despite many assertions, there is no convincing evidence that CMV is associated with a specific form of glomerulonephritis.

Human immunodeficiency virus (HIV)

- A variety of renal lesions occur in patients with HIV infection, even when full-blown AIDS has not developed. Some of these lesions may be a consequence of associated infectious illnesses or drug therapy.
- There does seem to be a specific HIV-associated nephropathy (HIVAN) found in HIV-positive patients.
- Although reported in all groups of HIV-positive patients, HIVAN is more common in African-American heterosexuals who are i.v. drug abusers (in some patients heroin nephropathy may coexist). It has also been found in infants infected by maternal transmission *in utero*.
- Clinical presentation is with sudden onset of severe nephrotic syndrome, with rapid deterioration to ESRF. Biopsy shows a focal and segmental glomerulosclerosis (FSGS), widespread tubuloreticular inclusions and tubular dilatation with protein casts.

Hantaviruses

- Haemorrhagic fever with renal syndrome (HFRS) is the name given to a number of related conditions occurring in response to infection with DNA viruses from the Hantavirus genus of the Bunyaviridae. The primary pathogenesis is likely to be immune complex-mediated vascular damage, rather than a direct cytopathic action on renal cells.

- HFRS is spread to humans from chronically infected wild rodents. The severity, prognosis and epidemiology of HFRS depends upon which particular serotype of the virus is implicated. HFRS primarily affects farmers, foresters, military personnel and those engaged in rural activities. Laboratory workers may also be affected.

- The most severe form occurs in East Asia following infection by the Hantaan serotype. Presentation is with high fever, abdominal and back pain, blurred vision, thirst, nausea and anorexia. Thrombocytopenia with haemorrhage into internal organs, hypotension and shock may occur. Oliguria is frequent, even in the absence of significant hypotension. ARF with haematuria and proteinuria occurs, followed by a diuretic recovery phase. A case fatality rate of about 5% is characteristic. This condition was formerly referred to as Korean haemorrhagic fever (KHF) and follows contact with the striped field mouse.

- A milder form occurs in western and central Europe, due to infection with the Puumala serotype. This follows contact with infected bank voles. There are usually no prodromal symptoms. High fever, lasting up to 7 days, occurs with signs of meningoencephalitis, abdominal pain, blurred vision and oliguric ARF. Haemorrhage and hypotension are much less marked than in the East Asian variant and recovery is more rapid. Case fatality rates of less than 0.5% have been reported. This condition is also referred to as nephropathica epidemica (NE).

- Illnesses of intermediate severity occur with infection by the Seoul serotype (carried by the Norwegian rat and predominantly a disease of urban areas) and the Maaji/Fornica serotype which is endemic in the Balkans.
- Renal biopsy findings are non-specific, with features of interstitial nephritis and interstitial haemorrhage in severe cases. Treatment is supportive and symptomatic, with most cases having a good prospect of recovery.
- Antibodies to Puumala virus are found in about 1.5% of blood donors in certain western European countries, suggesting that sub-clinical infection is common.

Other viruses

- BK and JC papovaviruses may be implicated in the pathogenesis of Balkan endemic nephropathy and are known to cause disease in renal transplant recipients.
- Renal failure is a common pre-terminal event in the now very uncommon yellow fever.
- Mumps virus, measles virus and herpes viruses have been reported, on a few occasions, to cause renal disease.

Further reading

Ko KW and Park HC (eds). Virus-related renal disease. *Kidney International*, 1991; Suppl. 35.

Related topics of interest

Focal segmental glomerulosclerosis (p. 77)
Membranous nephropathy (p. 117)
Post-infectious and mesangiocapillary glomerulonephritis (p. 139)

INDEX

Acetazolamide, 65, 67
Acetoacetic acid, 1
Acid–base disorders, **1–6**
Acidaemia, 2
Acidosis, 1, 33, 50, 52, 65
   diabetic ketoacidosis, 3
   metabolic, 3, 64
   renal tubular, *see* Renal tubular acidosis
   respiratory, 3, 5, 6, 64
   uraemic, 3
Acquired cystic disease, **225–226**
Acute renal failure, **7–10, 11–17**, 57, 58, 59,
   90, 98, 102, 105, 113, 135, 139, 142,
   151, 152, 171, 177, 199, 200, 210, 213,
   230, 237
Acute tubular necrosis, **7–10**, 57, 61, 67, 178,
   214
Acyclovir, 57
Addison's disease, 56, 195
Adynamic bone, 183–184
Agenesis, renal, 41
Alcohol, 22
Aldosterone, 64
Alkalosis, 52
   metabolic, 4, 5, 67
   respiratory, 6
Allopurinol, 9, 57, 114, 234
Alport's syndrome, 22, 85, **129**, 153
Aluminium, 158, 160, 182, 183
Amiloride, 66
Aminoaciduria, 113, 192, 194
Aminoglycosides, 13, 57, 59, 68
Ammonia, 2
Amphotericin, 57, **59**, 76, 194
Amylase, 50
Amyloidosis, 35, 163, **167–170**, 175, 193,
   194, 196
   dialysis-related, 92
Anaemia, 22, 33, **158–162**, 224, 226
Analgesic nephropathy, **18–20**, 32, 57, 175,
   195, 227
Anderson-Fabry disease, 131
Angiography, renal, 14, 37, 112, 198
Angiomyolipomas, 131
Angioplasty, 199
Angiotensin, 102, 209
Angiotensin converting enzyme, 231

Angiotensin converting enzyme inhibitors, 14,
   29, 33, 34, 47, 57, **58**, 66, 78, 80, 119,
   142, 147, 174, 195, 197, 199, 204, 211
Anion gap, 3, 4
Ankylosing spondylitis, 105
Antegrade pyelography, 127
Anticoagulation, 85, 90, 96, 119, 200
Antidiuretic hormone, **70**, 72, 102
   syndrome of inappropriate ADH secretion,
   75
Anti-glomerular basement membrane
   antibody, 14
   disease, 13, 129, **152–153**, 189
Antineutrophil cytoplasmic antibody, 14, 83,
   149–152
Antinuclear antibodies, 14, 83
Antiphospholipid antibody syndrome, **173**,
   213
Antithymocyte globulin, 188
Aquaporin, 71
Arteriovenous fistula, 90
Ascites, 55, 122
Aspirin, 142, 173, 199, 211
Atheromatous embolism, *see* Cholesterol
   embolism
Automated peritoneal dialysis, *see* Peritoneal
   dialysis
Autosomal dominant polycystic kidney
   disease 22, **26–30**, 32, 85, 203
Azathioprine, 79, 106, 108, 152, 172,
   187–188, 213

β-adrenergic agonists, 64, 66
β-blockers, 47, 65, 205
β-lactam antibiotics, 57, 114, 222
Balkan nephropathy, 115, 227, 238
Bartter's syndrome, 5, 67
Bence-Jones proteinuria, 144, 177, 178
Benign prostatic hyperplasia, 125
Berger's disease, *see* Glomerulonephritis, IgA
Bicarbonate, plasma, 3
Bio-incompatibility, 95
Bisphonates, *see* Diphosphonates
Bladder cancer, *see* Urothelial malignancy
Blood group antigens, 99, 220
Brain stem death, 186
Bronchiectasis, 168